the natural child

The fruits of good mothering and early nurture are among the greatest blessings a person can have in life. In offering these to their babies, mothers and fathers are setting the pattern of relationships which can be creative, mutually rewarding, and last for the rest of their lives. From her rich experience as a psychologist, parent and educator, Jan Hunt has lucidly described how this may be achieved with joy and satisfaction. I commend the wisdom she has distilled in this book to parents who wish the best for their children and themselves. Few things are more important for the healthy future of life on our planet.

— Dr. Peter Cook, consultant child psychiatrist, and author of *Early Child Care: Infants & Nations at Risk*

Jan Hunt is a most diligent, energetic, and well-informed person with regard to children's issues. She is one of the few people who understands and can write about the real needs of children as opposed to the rationalized needs of parents in relation to their children. Moreover, she can do this in an engaging fashion that does not put parents off. For the sake of children everywhere, I hope that her book is widely read and taken to heart.

— Dr. Elliott Barker, Director, Canadian Society for the Prevention of Cruelty to Children

The author... is a firm believer in the importance of empathizing with children and responding to them with concern, protection, and tenderness. Her essays are some of the finest examples in print of how a nurturing attitude to children can lead to appropriate and sane solutions to most of the common conflicts between children and their caretakers.

— James Kimmel, clinical psychologist, and author of *Whatever Happened to Mother*

A great book! Jan Hunt gives parents that most important advice in child-rearing: show your child respect. But she goes one step further: she gives example after example — a whole book full of how to do it. And therein lies the strength of *The Natural Child*: the reader gets a look at how to show respect in numerous situations. By the end of the book, the "how" in other situations has become self-evident. Follow her suggestions, and discover how rewarding it is to show respect to children. Does it work? I am a grandmother now, and I am often touched when I see the gentle, loving respect my grandson is receiving.

— Tine Thevenin, author of *The Family Bed* and
Mothering and Fathering

The Natural Child: Parenting from the Heart is an important resource for parents and professionals in all areas of child development. Jan Hunt's essays are full of warmth and empathy for all children, and give parents tools for making important decisions about how they want to raise their children. Our organization promotes loving, empathic parenting to create a peaceful world, and we firmly believe that this will be the most important message for society in the 21st Century. We will recommend that Attachment Parenting International's support groups add *The Natural Child* to their group libraries.

— Barbara Nicholson and Lysa Parker, co-founders,
Attachment Parenting International, "Parenting for a Peaceful World"

Jan Hunt's *The Natural Child* is a provocative, insightful, and useful book. It is excellent for anyone who is wary of conventional child-rearing practices and who seeks support and ideas for living and learning with children in new ways.

— Patrick Farenga, President of John Holt Associates, publisher of
Growing Without Schooling

the natural child
parenting from the heart

JAN HUNT

Foreword by Peggy O'Mara

NEW SOCIETY PUBLISHERS

Cataloguing in Publication Data:
A catalog record for this publication is available from the National Library of Canada.

"Lonely Cages!" combines material from two articles available on the Natural Child Project website: "Let's Abolish Cribs!" and "Ten Reasons to Sleep Next to Your Child at Night." "It Shouldn't Hurt to be a Child" combines material from "It Shouldn't Hurt to be a Child" and "Ten Reasons Not to Hit Your Kids," also available on the Natural Child website.

Cover design by Greg Green. Cover image: © 2001 Eyewire.
Printed in Canada by Friesens.

New Society Publishers acknowledges the support of the Government of Canada through the Book Publishing Industry Development Program (BPIDP) for our publishing activities, and the assistance of the Province of British Columbia through the British Columbia Arts Council.

BRITISH
COLUMBIA
ARTS COUNCIL
Supported by the Province of British Columbia

Paperback ISBN: 0-86571-440-1

Inquiries regarding requests to reprint all or part of *The Natural Child* should be addressed to New Society Publishers at the address below.

To order directly from the publishers, please add $4.50 shipping to the price of the first copy, and $1.00 for each additional copy (plus GST in Canada). Send check or money order to:

New Society Publishers
P.O. Box 189, Gabriola Island, BC V0R 1X0, Canada

New Society Publishers' mission is to publish books that contribute in fundamental ways to building an ecologically sustainable and just society, and to do so with the least possible impact on the environment, in a manner that models this vision. We are committed to doing this not just through education, but through action. We are acting on our commitment to the world's remaining ancient forests by phasing out our paper supply from ancient forests worldwide. This book is one step towards ending global deforestation and climate change. It is printed on acid-free paper that is **100% old growth forest-free** (100% post-consumer recycled), processed chlorine free, and printed with vegetable based, low VOC inks. For further information, or to browse our full list of books and purchase securely, visit our website at: www.newsociety.com

NEW SOCIETY PUBLISHERS   www.newsociety.com

The best way to make children good
is to make them happy.

— Oscar Wilde

Dedication

To Jason, who has
brought joy, play, and
love into my life since
the day he was born.

Contents

Foreword

Peggy O'Mara
Mothering Magazine

JAN HUNT TELLS THE TRUTH about the real nature of children. Many terms are popular today — attachment, natural, empathic — to describe a way of parenting that is really not new at all. Being with children in the way that these terms describe is what parents all over the world have done since the beginning of time. Jan points the way for us today. The cultural voices of fear tell us to distrust the neediness and dependency that children so naturally express. It is an acceptance of this neediness and dependency that Jan speaks about so eloquently. By modeling this acceptance, she makes it easier for us to accept our children and ourselves as well.

It's not often that I open a book and find that I have as much in common with the author's point of view as I do with Jan's. I often check the index of books for references to breastfeeding, co-sleeping, discipline, attachment, and other topics dear to my heart and seldom find the compatibility that I feel when I read *The Natural Child*. We have the same understanding about the nature of the child and both want to remedy the misunderstandings about children in modern culture.

When we make up new names like attachment parenting for old ways, it is because we are looking for more enduring wisdom than adversarial customs offer. We know that the bliss we feel parenting from the heart means that it is right. In regards to our children, it is not only wisdom we seek, but also an acknowledgement of our participation in a deeper process.

The great anthropologist, Margaret Mead, studied tribes all over the world. She said that the most violent tribes were those that withheld touch in infancy. To me, it is very simple. The propensity to act aggressively is related to unmet needs. When we objectify our babies and manipulate their legitimate needs to meet our own comfort level or prescription for living, we may unknowingly put them at risk. We can instead choose to surrender to the mystery of our baby's needs and the surprises he or she brings just as we would surrender and adapt to the surprises brought by new love. A baby is our new love.

Can we choose love by accepting our baby's legitimate human needs and responding to them with an open heart? This requires that we trust our babies and ultimately that we trust ourselves. Each of us is an original. We are equipped for the job even though we are still learning how to use our equipment. Most of our decisions as parents are more about our state of mind than about the particulars of the situation. When we choose from love we act very differently than when we act from fear.

Jan tells it like it is. Children and adults are not different. We have the same feelings. Children who are disciplined with love respond lovingly. Parents are not perfect, but we can continually recognize the critical importance of how we behave toward our children. Crying is the language of babies. Co-sleeping is safe and smart. Children need to be involved in the problem-solving of the family. Punishment interferes with the bond between parent and child. Children have a natural love of learning and do not have to be coerced. Learning "disabilities" may be learning differences. Children deserve to be acknowledged in public. Children deserve to be treated with respect.

These shared beliefs are why Jan and I are so compatible. We've never met and compared notes. And while we have both been influenced by many of the same people, there are simply many common conclusions that stem from trusting and respecting children. It sounds easy, but we all know that what I describe is a lifetime journey. Many of us have been raised in cultures and families where control is highly valued. Our children are often our first teachers in this regard. In learning to trust them, we learn that we can be trusted as well.

It is the potential limitlessness of simply trusting our children that frightens parents. We ask how we can maintain order and harmony in the household without control, without punishment. As Jan will so aptly teach, the household based on empathy, compassion and cooperation will have an inherent discipline that does not have to be enforced by punishment. It is enforced by love.

This book is about simple principles that can take a lifetime to learn. As the parent of adult children, I can attest to the helpfulness of breastfeeding, co-sleeping, home schooling, discipline without punishment and other trusting choices. All of these choices are implicit in the egalitarian relationship that I hope to have with my children. They are my equals, my teachers and my beloved ones. I try to remember this when I interact with them. Jan's book will help you remember too.

Acknowledgments

I AM INDEBTED TO MY SON, Jason Hunt, who edited and printed the initial manuscript for this book with extraordinary dedication and care. My words are much clearer thanks to his insightful attention to detail and generous donation of time to this project.

A sincere thank-you to Marcus Hunt, Denise Green, Bonnie Gonzales and Elisabeth Hallett for their careful reading of my articles, creative suggestions, and personal encouragement over the years. Many thanks to Susan Buckley for inspiring me to follow my dreams.

Thanks to Susannah Sheffer of Holt Associates, whose early publication of my letters and articles in *Growing Without Schooling* helped launch my writing career, and to Wendy Priesnitz for requesting my parenting column and running it in *Natural Life* for nine years. Thank you to Peggy O'Mara, *Mothering* editor and publisher, for her continued enthusiasm for my work and for her kindness in writing this book's foreword despite her busy schedule.

Thank you also to David Albert for his encouragement and enthusiasm, and his assistance in finding a publisher for this book.

And a very special thank-you to Chris Plant, Audrey McClellan and the staff at New Society Publishers for recognizing the importance of helping parents to treat their children with trust and compassion, and for being a living example of these qualities in all of my interactions with them.

Introduction

T*HE NATURAL CHILD* IS A collection of essays on parenting and education that I wrote between 1988 and the
present. Many of the essays appeared in the Canadian publication *Natural Life*, to which I contributed a parenting
column from 1989 to 1999 (<www.life.ca/nl/>). Others
have been included on the Natural Child Project website
<www.naturalchild.org> since 1996.

I wrote the essays to help parents and future parents
understand the critical importance of treating their children with dignity, respect, understanding, and
compassion from infancy into adulthood. I hope to
inspire parents toward a new way of being with their children that allows for a mutually trusting and loving
relationship based on respectful, gentle guidance and
emotional support.

This approach has been called "attachment parenting"
or "empathic parenting." It is often considered to be New
Age, but it is in fact age-old. Many of the practices that I
recommend in this book were the norm for thousands of
generations and have only been questioned within the last
hundred years or less.

Empathic parenting, to put it simply, is believing what we know in our heart to be true. If we follow our hearts, we trust the child in these ways:

- We understand that all children are doing the very best they can at every given moment.
- We trust that though children may be small in size, they deserve to have their needs taken seriously.
- We know that it is unrealistic to expect a child to behave perfectly at all times.
- We recognize that "bad behavior" is the child's attempt to communicate an important need in the best way she can.
- We learn to look beneath the child's outward behavior to understand what he is thinking and feeling.
- We see that in a very beautiful way, our child teaches us what love is.

Children raised with love and compassion will be free to use their time as adults in meaningful and creative ways, rather than expressing their childhood hurts in ways that harm themselves or others. If adults have no need to deal with the past, they can live fully in the present.

The educator John Holt once said that everything he wrote could be summed up in two words: "trust children." This is the most precious gift we can give as parents.

I believe that through empathic parenting the world can become a more peaceful and a more humane place, where every child can grow to adulthood with a generous capacity for empathy and trust. Our society has no more urgent task.

Jan Hunt
October 2001

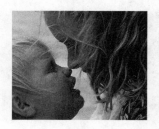

PARENTING WITH EMPATHY AND TRUST

"Getting It" About Children

WHAT DOES IT MEAN to "get it" about children? This concept, which I refer to regularly in my work as a counselor and writer, seems to be a "zero or one" condition; people either get it or they don't. They either understand that children are human beings who deserve to be treated like human beings — or they just don't get it. Unfortunately, there are many people in our society who don't get it. And surprisingly, this includes many mental health professionals.

What does it mean when someone *doesn't* get it? It means they have succumbed to the notion that children are basically different from adults. It means that they think children operate on vastly different principles of behavior than adults do. They must think this, because no adults would *improve* their behavior by being hit, insulted, criticized, yelled at, or punished in any way. Adults behave as well as they are treated — everyone knows that. Why, then, does everyone not know the same is true for children? Why is it assumed that children will behave better if they are punished? Obviously they may change their behavior due to fear, but as psychologist and author Marshall Rosenberg

reminds us, there are two questions we need to ask ourselves
when we want to change a child's behavior:

> *Two questions help us see why we are unlikely to get*
> *what we want by using punishment .... The first ques-*
> *tion is:* What do I want this person to do that's dif-
> ferent from what he or she is currently doing? *If we*
> *ask only this first question, punishment may seem effec-*
> *tive because the threat or exercise of punitive force may*
> *well influence the person's behavior. However, with the*
> *second question, it becomes evident that punishment*
> *isn't likely to work:* What do I want this person's rea-
> sons to be for doing what I'm asking?
>
> *We seldom address the latter question, but when*
> *we do, we soon realize that ... punishment damages*
> *good will and self-esteem and shifts our attention*
> *from the intrinsic value of an action to external con-*
> *sequences. Blaming and punishing fail to contribute*
> *to the motivations we would like to inspire in others.*[1]

Dr. Rosenberg is a psychologist who "gets it," clearly
and completely. Yet there are many who do not. There are
many who would believe that Dr. Rosenberg's description
may be accurate for adults, but not for children. Yet if children are indeed so different from adults, on exactly what day
of their life do they suddenly change their operating principles? On the morning of their 18th birthday? Their 21st?
No one can answer that question, because there is no such
transition. Human beings of all ages operate on the very
same principles: they behave well when treated well by
another, and they respond by wanting to treat that person
well in return. They behave poorly when deliberately hurt

by another, and they react with anger and resentment and a wish to hurt that person in return. It makes no difference that mistreatment is rationalized in the parent's mind as being "for their own good" — to the child, such motivation is irrelevant. All they see is the action itself.

If we don't get it, and we believe that children have strange and different principles of behavior, then parenting is much more complicated. We are forever guessing what to do. Do we count to five or ten before spanking? Do we give two minutes of time-out or five? Do we ground our teenager for a day or a week? Do we apologize for our mistakes or do we present a perfect front to our child?

> *Every child is no less a human being than we are.*

If we do get it, if we understand that children have the same operating principles, the same human nature that we all have, it becomes a simple matter to predict how they will respond to our actions. All we need to do is ask ourselves how *we* would respond in the same situation. Parenting becomes a relatively simple matter of applying the Golden Rule. As Dr. Elliott Barker, director of the Canadian Society for the Prevention of Child Abuse, puts it so eloquently:

> *Children who have their needs met early by loving parents are subjected totally and thoroughly to the most severe form of "discipline" conceivable:* they don't do what you don't want them to do because they love you so much!
>
> *If you haven't cluttered the airwaves between you and your child with a thousand stupid "don'ts" over*

> *your Royal Doulton china, or not eating their dessert*
> *before the main course, or not finishing their spinach,*
> *or not doing this or that, then those few situations*
> *where it really matters because of safety and impro-*
> *priety don't need anything approaching the*
> *connotation of "discipline" to ensure appropriate*
> *behavior.*[2]

Every child is no less a human being than we are. They deserve to be treated with dignity, respect, understanding, and compassion. When they are treated this way, everyone benefits.

The Importance of Empathic Parenting

> Any person who abuses his children has himself
> been severely traumatized in his childhood...
> there is no reason for child abuse other than the
> repression of the abuse and confusion once
> suffered by the abuser himself.
>
> — Alice Miller[1]

HOW DOES AN ABUSED CHILD overcome painful experiences enough to give his own children more love than he himself was given? Are such children, as they reach adulthood, doomed to repeat an endless cycle of anger, abuse, and retaliation? Or are there ways to stop the cycle and learn more empathic, responsive ways of treating children?

While it is likely that hurtful parents were themselves hurt in childhood, repetition of this pattern is not inevitable. Some abused children grow up determined to give their own children the childhood they missed. My father, who was sometimes beaten and sometimes belittled by his father, expressed it as the desire "to give my children a better life than I had."

The simplicity of this statement is an illusion. It actually encompasses two complex steps: first, the parent must gain an awareness that he or she did indeed experience abuse in childhood. This is the most difficult step, because abusive experiences of childhood are so painful that we suppress them. They may thus become unavailable to us even when we feel ready to confront our emotional limitations. As Dr. Miller explains, "Many people can scarcely remember the torments of their childhood because they have learned to regard them as a justified punishment for their own 'badness' and also because a child must repress painful events in order to survive." However, it is not inevitable that every abused child become an abuser himself, "if, during childhood, he had the chance — be it only once — to encounter someone who offered him something other than pedagogy and cruelty: a teacher, an aunt, a neighbor, a sister, a brother. It is only through the experience of being loved and cherished that the child can ever discern cruelty as such, be aware of it, and resist it."

Awareness is not enough, though, to stop the cycle of abuse. The second step toward this goal is that the parents must learn new ways of relating to children, ways that they may have seldom, if ever, witnessed as children themselves. How can such parents learn to treat their own children with dignity and respect?

Dr. Elliott Barker recommends four critical steps that all prospective parents can take to raise emotionally healthy children, "no matter how inadequate their own past experience of nurturing has been."[2]

1. **A positive birthing experience.** As Dr. Barker explains, "If both parents are present at the birth, and there is a positive birthing experience, the mother and father are very likely to fall in love with their baby ... the hard work of looking after their child feels much less like hard work; they're obsessed with how wonderful their baby is."

2. **Extended breastfeeding.** "Breastfeeding until the child no longer requires it is another of those things a mother can do which will cause other good things to happen ... as if by magic," according to Dr. Barker. "Breastfeeding keeps you in love with your child. Extended breastfeeding can help the mother - infant attachment survive rough times which might otherwise lead to emotional unavailability and detachment."

3. **Minimal separations and consistency of caregivers.** According to pediatrician William Sears, only the parent "is perfectly attuned to the child's needs. Being away from [the child] during stressful times deprives him of his most valuable support and also deprives you of a chance to further cement your friendship .... Babies learn to accept unfulfilled needs, but at the cost of lowered self-esteem and the capacity to trust."[3]

4. **Careful spacing of children.** According to Dr. Barker, "it requires an enormous amount of time and energy on the part of both parents to adequately nurture one child under the age of three. Spacing children is one important thing that parents can do to prevent the exhaustion that

occurs when well-intentioned parents take on the very difficult task of trying to meet the emotional needs of closely spaced children."

These four steps can have a profound effect on the entire family. Not only do they establish the capacity to love and trust within the child, but they also help the parents to heal from the pain of their own childhood. By establishing a close bond of love and trust between parent and child, these steps can halt the cycle of abuse in one generation. Dr. Miller assures us that "it is absolutely impossible for someone who has grown up in an environment of honesty, respect, and affection ever to feel driven to torment a weaker person .... He has learned very early on that it is right and proper to provide the small, helpless creature with protection and guidance; this knowledge, stored at that early stage in his mind and body, will remain effective for the rest of his life." Such a child will grow up with a profound and unwavering conviction that it is wrong to hurt another human being.

Unfortunately, many new parents are unaware of these four critical steps, especially if they never experienced unconditional love and trust in their childhood. The relentless cycle of abuse can be stopped by means of educational programs that emphasize the four steps of empathic parenting, new legislation that gives children the protection they need and deserve, and the loving treatment of children by those who interact with families.

In Scandinavia, there are laws prohibiting child abuse — not only physical and sexual assault, but also spanking and bullying. These laws do not carry penalties; they are intended to raise public awareness of the legitimate needs

> *... the capacity to love and trust, once established within a child, can transfer down through the generations ...*

and rights of children. Will such legislation be effective, when all else has failed? Dr. Miller believes that "every human being caught in a trap will search for a way out. And at heart he is glad and grateful if he is shown a way out that does not lead to guilt or to the destruction of his own children."

Fortunately the capacity to love and trust, once established within a child, can transfer down through the generations as readily as can mistrust and cruelty. Dr. Miller assures us that "it is quite simply not true that human beings must continue compulsively to injure their children .... Injuries can heal and need not be passed on, provided they are not ignored. It is perfectly possible ... to be open to the messages from our children that can help us never again to destroy life but rather to protect it and allow it to blossom."

Nature or Nurture?

IN JUDITH RICH HARRIS'S BOOK *The Nurture Assumption*, she makes the argument that peers, and not parents, are most responsible for who children become.

In response, consider this excerpt from an article on the origins of teenage rebellion, "The Relationship Between Feelings and Behavior," by Dr. Sidney Craig:

If we want our children to spend time with us, to like us, to confide in us, to value some of the things we value, and to try to make us happy (for example, by refraining from the use of dangerous drugs), we must behave toward them in ways that create feelings of love toward us rather than feelings of dislike or anger. We cannot reasonably expect to receive "good" behavior from our children unless we create "good" feelings in them.[1]

Because it is so painful for an adult to recognize and remember the pain of betrayal in infancy and early childhood, self-deception is likely. In her landmark article "Childhood Trauma," Alice Miller explains:

Information about the cruelty suffered during childhood remains stored in the brain in the form of unconscious memories. For a child, conscious experience of such treatment is impossible. If children are not to break down completely under the pain and the fear, they must repress that knowledge. But the unconscious memories of the child who has been neglected and maltreated, even before he has learned to speak, drive the adult to reproduce those repressed scenes over and over again in the attempt to liberate himself from the fears that cruelty has left with him.[2]

Early childhood is the starting point for all love and for all cruelty in later years. To the degree that infants or children have been given compassion, they will pass it on to others in the future. There is a Swedish saying, *man far den respekt man ger:* "One gets the respect one gives." Unfortunately, the converse is also true. When we give disrespect (including all forms of punishment) to a child, we breed disrespect, anger, and retaliatory impulses within that child that will inevitably be passed on to others later.

Compassionate early parenting is like a well-built boat, protecting the child from the sea of all subsequent disappointments, temptations, frustrations, and sorrows. Blaming teenage crime on peer pressure (or video games, movies, music, clothing, the Internet, the media, or anything else in current culture) is like blaming a storm for overturning a child's poorly built boat. We know that there will always be storms in our children's lives. There will always be temptations, disappointments, sorrows, even tragedies. Their ability to cope with these events is what really matters. Do they have a strong enough boat, or do they have a boat with holes? Do they have any boat at all, or have they been put to sea without protection? And when they drown, do we blame the wind and the rain, the wake of passing motorboats, and the clutching hands of their boatless peers, or do we start building better boats for all of our children?

Let me use my son Jason as an example. Because he has been treated with love, compassion, and trust from birth, he is riding over the sea of life in a very sturdy boat.

A happy childhood lasts forever.

I find it difficult to imagine any circumstance or experience that would cause him to commit an inhumane action. He would simply withstand efforts by his peers to lead him in this direction. He would also put every effort into helping his peers have their relevant emotional needs met in a more sane and healthy way. I've seen him do this.

Because of the pain of recognizing the hurt and disappointment in our own childhood, we'll blame anything else to avoid feeling that sorrow. But the truth is as simple as this familiar slogan: A happy childhood lasts forever.

Tough Love

A RECENT NEWSPAPER STORY described parents who deliberately embarrassed their child at a mall by screaming at him and striking him. When one of the bystanders objected, the parents said they were "just using Tough Love."

"Tough Love" was originally intended for adult drug addicts, not for young children still learning about life. As used by the parents at the mall, Tough Love only teaches a child the harmful and illogical lesson that deliberately hurting another human being is supposedly "an act of love." Children instinctively know that this mangled definition of love makes no sense. But when this lesson is repeated often enough, they begin to believe it. A child who learns to associate love with pain grows up emotionally crippled, confusing cruelty with love and sadism with intimacy.

Parents who use Tough Love should remember that "the proof of the pudding is in the eating." Adolf Hitler was often humiliated and harshly disciplined in childhood, while the young Albert Einstein was consistently treated with gentleness, kindness, and patience. His mother was often accused of "spoiling" him. Fortunately, however, she ignored those warnings. As an adult, Hitler expressed the anguish and pain of those years in ways that brought misery and suffering to millions. By comparison, Einstein became not only one of the world's greatest scientists, but also a most gentle, caring man, deeply concerned about social issues.

These are extreme examples, of course, but there is no doubt in my mind that there is a close, direct correlation between the degree of punishment in childhood and later difficulties in adulthood, just as there is between loving parenting and later health and happiness.

Punishment, threats, and humiliation never achieve long-term goals because they provoke anger, create resentment, and diminish the bond between parent and child. Punishment interferes with the child's opportunity to learn from direct experience, which ideally should be unencumbered by fear and pain. As the educator John Holt warned, "When we make a child afraid, we stop learning dead in its tracks."

According to the mother in the newspaper story, her child was being punished because he forgot to flush a toilet in a public restroom; but what this child learned from the example set by his parents, and by those bystanders who did not intervene on his behalf, likely had nothing to do with bathroom hygiene. He learned that it is right and proper to cause and then to ignore a "loved" one's suffering. He learned that even those who claim to love us can hurt us. In fact, he probably learned that it is foolish to believe people who claim to love us and that it is dangerous to allow ourselves to be close to others. His parents' harsh and unfeeling treatment taught him that the world is a mean and dangerous place. Such beliefs form the worst possible foundation for life. They are the attitudes toward life and self that are most likely to induce angry behavior in childhood and lead to a life of emotionally impoverished, self-centered, and ultimately futile attempts to meet critical needs — needs that should have been met in childhood.

The boy's parents are, in all likelihood, well-meaning, and probably learned their teaching methods from their own parents. They think they are teaching their son to do the right thing and to grow to be a responsible adult. Ironically, their behavior is likely to accomplish just the opposite: a U.S. Army study found that good experiences, not painful ones, best prepare a child for adult responsibilities.[1]

> *good experiences, not painful ones, best prepare a child for adult responsibilities.*

What these parents did to their child is clearly abusive. Unfortunately, North American laws are not as clear about what constitutes emotional abuse as are laws that exist in many other countries. In Sweden, for example, it is illegal not only to hit a child, but also to bully him.

A follow-up letter to the newspaper suggested that the parents be required to wear signs saying "I am a child abuser." Unfortunately, such a sign can be translated as "I am a former abused child." And so it goes through the generations — until schools teach enlightened parenting skills, and until new child abuse laws are written that clearly promote the respectful treatment of children.

The letter writer suggested that the bystanders should have called the police. Perhaps, but there are a few other calls to be made. Call legislators to strengthen laws against emotional child abuse. Call school superintendents and remind them that learning positive parenting skills is more valuable than memorizing dates of historical battles. Call judges, who need to understand the link between child-hood punishment and adult crime so they can stop recommending "more discipline" and start prescribing classes for abusive parents. Call expectant parents and remind them of the underlying principles of behavior: that children reflect the treatment they receive, and that chil-dren are human beings who deserve to be treated with dignity and respect. Call newspaper editors and tell them that articles teaching compassionate parenting are infinitely more important than stories about men throwing balls through hoops, even if sports coverage sells more papers. Call those adults who are lucky enough to be parents and who have had difficulty adjusting to that role. Gently sug-gest that if they have had a painful childhood, perhaps they might consider counseling so that the cycle of child abuse can be stopped now.

It's not surprising that a child with "tough" parents would be so preoccupied with painful feelings that he might forget to flush a toilet. He'll probably forget a lot of things, but what he'll remember is that it is dangerous to trust other people, acceptable to ignore the suffering of children, and less painful to live a life of loneliness and isolation than to risk being hurt any further.

To love a child means to treat him or her with respect, patience, gentleness, and compassion, in a way that is con-sistent with the Golden Rule. Tough Love is tough, all right, but it has nothing to do with love.

Confessions of a Proud Mom

MY SON IS 15 and has brought me nothing but ...

Trouble?

I thought you would say that! No, my son is 15 and has brought me nothing but joy.

You're kidding! How did you do that?

I am proud of my son but, unfortunately, I cannot take personal credit. His father and I were simply fortunate enough, after some missteps at the start, to read insightful parenting books and magazines, and to explore parenting issues with knowledgeable and compassionate friends. Today he is the most caring, thoughtful, and generous person I know.

Tell me, please! What did you do?

Well, we did everything we were told by society not to do. He slept next to us, breast-fed for several years, was never punished, threatened, bullied, or teased, and was allowed to express anger as well as happiness ....

Oh, you spoiled him?

Well, let's examine that word. The dictionary defines "spoil" as "to cause to demand or expect too much by overindulgence." In my dictionary, this is the third definition. It mirrors the common usage of this word in our society and it denotes a cause and effect: overindulgence, it says, causes spoiling. But is this belief true? Or does this definition merely represent a widespread misunderstanding of the true nature of children's behavior? A definition that would be accurate in terms of the way children actually learn and react is the first one listed: "to damage or injure, to destroy."

What actually spoils a child, what actually damages, injures, and destroys vital qualities in the child, are the other choices of parental behavior: punishment, separation, and rejection. These experiences spoil a child's inborn sense of trust, capacity to love, creativity, and potential for joy. Robbing a child of these treasures is surely one of the most harmful acts a human can perform.

Where can I find the kind of information that helped you?

Read *Mothering, The Compleat Mother,* and *Empathic Parenting.* Meet with caring mothers in La Leche League and other breast-feeding support groups. Talk with midwives. Read books by Alice Miller, Joseph Chilton Pearce, Tine Thevenin, and John Holt. Listen to what your heart tells you. Truly believe that your baby will let you know what is right ... and what is wrong.

How can a baby tell me this?

Babies come into the world with perfect love and trust. They do not suspect, mistrust, play mind games, doubt motives, or in any way cloud communication unless and until this trust is betrayed by such painful experiences as punishment, rejection, and parent-child separation. A baby's smiles and tears are the most potent form of communication on this planet.

What about the mistakes I've already made?

There are no perfect parents. While we have all made mistakes, punishing ourselves is no more effective or reasonable than punishing our children. Loving ourselves, and understanding that we have done as well as we could have with the information and inner strength we had at that moment, is as important as loving and understanding our children. We can put forth the love that we feel, recognize the critical importance of parenting, and continue to discover compassionate ways of relating to the children we are blessed with.

What are the most important things a parent should know?

Two things. First, our society assumes that children and adults operate on two separate and distinct codes of behavior. As adults, we know that we behave at our best when we are treated with kindness, patience, and understanding. Yet we presume that children behave best when they are threatened, punished, and humiliated. If we try to pinpoint the age at which the mysterious transformation from "children's principles of behavior" to "adult principles of behavior" occurs, we are at a loss, because there is no such transformation. There is no difference between how children and adults behave: we all behave as well as we are treated.

Secondly, a child's misbehavior provides an opportunity for parents to give the child important validation for her feelings and gentle instruction about life. For example, a child who has just hit a friend can be told: "I can see how angry you are. You really wanted that toy yourself, but it's Joey's turn now. It's OK to be angry but it's not OK to hit him. What would you like to do instead while you're waiting your turn?" With this type of response, the child receives accurate feedback about friendship and learns by example how to respond to an angry person with patience and empathy.

we all behave as well as we are treated.

If instead the parent introduces punishment, the opportunity to learn from the situation is lost, because the child's attention is taken away from the matter at hand and drawn instead into feelings of humiliation and anger, and fantasies of revenge. Little is learned about how to behave the next time the situation arises.

Finally, superficial "good behavior" obtained through threats and punishment can only take place until the child is old enough to fight back. But if trust, kindness, and empathy are kept intact within the child from birth and strengthened by parental examples of those qualities, they will last a lifetime.

I see. It's all a matter of trusting children, of recognizing that children may be less experienced and smaller than we are, but that they deserve to be treated with dignity and respect as much as adults do. From newborns to centenarians, all human beings behave as well as they are treated.

Memories of a Loving Father

This article is dedicated with love and gratitude to Nathan Baron (1903 — 1990).

M Y FATHER GREW UP IN A large Russian immigrant family in northern Ohio. There were eleven children in the family and numerous relatives nearby.

Dad often reminisced about his early family life. He once described a typical day at home: his mother kept a list of transgressions, and when his father arrived home from work, he would take a strap to each of the offenders. His mother would intervene only to the point of pleading "Not the head! Not the head!" My father never labeled this treatment "child abuse," but he knew it was wrong to treat children in this way.

To help with family finances, my dad had a job selling newspapers on the street starting at age eight; he was not allowed to return home until he had sold all his papers. He would probably not have called this child abuse either.

Dad often spoke of his deep desire to give his children the childhood that he had missed. He never hit his own children, and although he sometimes misunderstood our intentions, he always tried to do what he believed was in our best interest. When I once asked him how he had been able to treat my brother and me better than his own father had treated him, he replied, simply, "I wanted my children to have a better life than I had." My father was a good example of a man who somehow found it in his heart to treat his own children with more compassion than he himself had received as a child.

I once asked my mother how Dad was able to be so loving despite having been punished so often by his father. Mom quickly replied, "Sarah. His sister Sarah protected him." I found it interesting that my mother, who had never studied the emotional origins of behavior, had this perceptive insight. I owe much to Sarah — and she herself must have been protected by someone. This is what gives me hope: love moves through the generations as readily as does pain.

Dad died in 1990, at the age of 87. For the last few years of his life he suffered from prostate cancer, poor vision, and frailty. He was nearly blind, somewhat deaf, and used a walker. Slender all his life, he had become painfully thin. A man who enjoyed more than 80 healthy, active years had been vanquished. But you would not have heard that from him. Just a few months before his death he would be as eagerly excited as a small child if we were going out for dinner. One day, during what turned out to be my last visit with him, he used a walker for the first time in my presence. I must have looked surprised, because he put his arm around me and whispered, "I don't really need this. I'm only using it to please your mother." After Dad died, I shared that memory with Mom. We marveled at the strength of his proud will, which not even cancer could break.

Although Dad lived into his late 80s, for me he will always be in his early 40s, so vivid and special are my memories of our times together when I was a small child. Though he was a hardworking and busy man, first as a traveling salesman and later as a retailer, he managed to spend enough time with me that I picture him always at home.

My most precious memories are those of our trips around the block — Dad walking, I on my tricycle. I must have been three or four. After we passed two corners, we could see the houses that backed against those on our own street, and I would get excited. Most of these houses were English Tudor style, while those on our block were typical American 1940s architecture of wood and brick. My excitement came not from seeing a different architectural style, but because Dad would pretend that this was England — not merely English architecture, but England itself! There I was at age three, a global traveler, visiting England every day. Dad always loved to travel, and he always believed in dreams.

Dad traveled often when I was small, but he made it clear that he deeply missed all of us when he was away from home. I had a collection of international dolls, dressed in various traditional costumes. Whenever Dad returned from a business trip, he would greet me with great excitement and pleasure and present me with a new doll. Yet it wasn't the dolls themselves that mattered to me, and I never felt that he was using gifts as a substitute for his presence. The dolls were simply his way of telling me that he had missed me and that he had thought of me while we were apart — a subtle message for a young child, but he managed to communicate it. He would describe in great detail his trip to the store, then tell me his reasons for having chosen that particular doll and a little about the country represented. His pleasure and delight in my happiness were obvious.

Dad had a wonderful sense of humor; he would instantly stop whatever he was doing if someone had a joke to share, and we laughed often in our family. Dad's favorite comedian was Jack Benny. Like Jack, every year on his birthday Dad would turn 39. When I actually *became* 39, he joked that we were now the same age. He gave me the precious gift of seeing humor in the most difficult situations.

Shortly before Dad died, I dreamed of his death. In my dream I felt deep sadness and complained to a friend, "But now I can't tell him any more jokes."

We seldom hear this when a man of his age dies, but it's true of my dad: "He was so young."

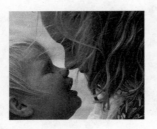

LIVING WITH A BABY

A Baby Cries: How Should
Parents Respond?

IMAGINE FOR A MOMENT THAT YOU have been abducted by alien beings on a spaceship and taken to a distant planet where you are surrounded by giant strangers whose language you do not speak. Two of those strangers take you under their care. You are entirely dependent on them for the satisfaction of all your needs: hunger, thirst, comfort, and — especially — reassurance that you are safe in this strange place. Then imagine that you are in pain or terribly thirsty or in need of emotional support, but your two attendants ignore your cries of distress. You are unable to get them to help you or to understand your needs. Now you have another problem, more serious than the first: you feel completely helpless and alone in an alien world.

No one likes to have their communication ignored. When it is ignored, this brings on feelings of helplessness and anger that inevitably damage the relationship. This response seems to be universally experienced by adults, and there is no reason to conclude that it is any different for babies and children. Few people would ignore an adult repeatedly saying, "Can you help me? I'm not feeling right." But a baby cannot make such a statement; he can only cry and cry until someone responds — or until he gives up in despair.

In modern western culture, we assume that crying is normal and unavoidable for babies. Yet for thousands of years, adults responded immediately and unquestioningly to a baby's cry. In societies where babies are carried close to the caregiver much of the day and night for the first several months, such crying is rare. And in contrast to what many in our society would expect, babies cared for in this way show self-sufficiency sooner than babies who do not receive such care.

children who have enjoyed the most loving care in infancy become the most secure and loving adults

In fact, research on early childhood experiences consistently shows that children who have enjoyed the most loving care in infancy become the most secure and loving adults, while those babies who have been forced into submissive behavior build up feelings of resentment and anger that may be expressed later in harmful ways.[1]

In spite of this research, most arguments for ignoring crying are based on fears of "spoiling" the baby. A typical baby-care brochure advises the parent to "let the baby handle it for a while."

Though infancy can be a challenging time for the parents, a baby is simply too young and inexperienced to "handle" the cause of the crying, whatever it may be. He cannot feed himself, change himself, or comfort himself in the way that nature intended. Clearly it is the parents' responsibility to meet their baby's needs for nurturing, security, and love; it is not the baby's responsibility to meet his parents' need for peace and solitude.

The baby-care pamphlet implies that if the parents give their baby an opportunity to become self-reliant, they are helping her to mature. But an infant is not capable of such maturity. True maturity reflects a strong foundation of emotional security that can only come about from the love and support of those closest to her during the earliest years.

In all innocence, a baby assumes that we, her parents, are correct — whatever we do is what we ought to be doing. If we do nothing, the baby can only conclude that she is unloved because she is unlovable. It is not within her capabilities to conclude that we are only busy, distracted, worried, misled by "experts," or simply inexperienced as parents. No matter how deeply we love our baby, she can only understand the outward manifestation of that love.

An immature person responds to stress in an immature way. A baby denied her birthright of comforting from her parents may respond by turning to ineffective self-stimulation (head-banging, rhythmic rocking, thumb-sucking, etc.) and emotional withdrawal from others. If her needs are routinely ignored, she may decide that loneliness and despair are preferable to risking further disappointment and rejection. Unfortunately, once a baby makes this decision it can become a permanent outlook on life, leading to an emotionally impoverished future. Many child-care professionals feel that parents who encourage self-satisfiers or substitute material objects for their own presence — teddy bears substituting for parents, strollers for arms, cribs for shared sleep, pacifiers for nursing, toys for parents' attention, music boxes for voices, formula for breast milk, wind-up swings for laps — have contributed to an age of materialistic acquisition, personal loneliness, and lack of emotional fulfillment.

Ignoring a baby's crying is like using earplugs to stop the distressing noise of a smoke detector. The smoke detector is meant to alert us to a serious matter that requires a response — and so is the cry of a baby. As Jean Liedloff wrote in *The Continuum Concept,* "A baby's cry is precisely as serious as it sounds."[2]

Stressful though it may be, infant crying should be seen not as a power struggle between parent and child, but as a gift from nature to ensure that all babies can grow to adulthood with a generous capacity for love and trust.

Ten Reasons to Respond to a Crying Child

1. A baby's first attempts to communicate cannot be in words, but can only be nonverbal. She cannot put happy feelings into words, but she can smile. She cannot put sad or angry feelings into words, but she can cry. If her smiles receive a response, but crying is ignored, she can receive the harmful message that she is loved and cared for only when she is happy. Children who continue to get this message through the years cannot feel truly loved and accepted.

2. If a child's attempts to communicate sadness or anger are routinely ignored, he cannot learn how to express those feelings in words. Crying must receive an appropriate and positive response so the child sees that all of his feelings are accepted. If his feelings are not accepted, and crying is ignored or punished, he receives the message

that sadness and anger are unacceptable, no matter how they are expressed. It is impossible for a child to understand that his expression of sadness or anger will be accepted once he is older and able to use appropriate words. A child can only communicate in ways available to him at a given time; a child can only accomplish what he has had a chance to learn. Every child is doing his best according to his age, experience, and present circumstances. It is surely unfair to punish a child for not doing more than he can do.

3. A child who has been given the message that her parents will only respond to her when she is "good" will begin to hide "bad" behavior and "bad" feelings from others and even from herself. She may become an adult who submerges "bad" emotions and is unable to communicate the full range of human feelings. Indeed, there are many adults who find it difficult to express anger, sadness, or other "bad" feelings in an appropriate way.

4. Anger that cannot be expressed in early childhood does not simply disappear. It becomes repressed and builds up over the years, until the child is unable to contain it any longer and is old enough to have lost his fear of physical punishment. When this container of anger is finally thrown open, parents can be shocked and perplexed. They have forgotten the hundreds or thousands of moments of frustration that have been filling this container over the years. The psychological principle that "frustration leads to aggression" is never more clearly demonstrated than in the final rebellion of a teenager. Parents need to understand how frustrating it can be for a child to feel "invisible" when his crying is ignored, or

to feel helpless and discouraged when his attempts to express his needs and feelings are misunderstood, ignored or punished.

5. We are all born knowing that each and every feeling we have is legitimate. We gradually lose that belief if only our "good" side brings a positive response. This is a tragedy, because it is only when we fully accept ourselves and others, regardless of mistakes, that we can have truly loving relationships. If we are not fully loved and accepted in childhood, we may never learn how that feels or how to communicate that acceptance to others, no matter how much therapy or reading or thinking we do. How much easier our lives would be if we simply received unconditional love throughout our early years!

6. Parents wondering whether to respond to crying might think about their own responses in similar situations. They may consider it appropriate to ignore a child's cries, yet feel intensely angry if their partner ignores attempts to have a conversation. Many in our society seem to believe that a person must be a certain age before she has the right to be heard. Yet what age would that be? Infants and children are not any less human just because they are small and helpless. If anything, the more helpless people are, the more they deserve our compassion, attention, and assistance.

7. If children are taught by example that helpless people deserve to be ignored, they can lose the compassion for others that all humans are born with. If, as helpless infants, their cries are ignored, they begin to believe that this is the appropriate response to those who are weaker than themselves. Without compassion, the stage is set for

later violence. Those who wonder why a violent criminal has no compassion for his victims need to consider where he lost that compassion. It does not disappear overnight. It is stolen, through unresponsive or punitive parenting, drop by drop, until it is gone. Loss of compassion is the greatest tragedy that can befall a child.

8. When a child learns by her parents' example that it is appropriate to ignore a child's cries, she will naturally treat her own child the same way unless there is some intervention from others. Inadequate parenting continues through the generations until fortunate circumstances come about to change this pattern. How much easier it would be if a parent learned in childhood how to treat his or her own child! Perhaps the cycle of inadequate parenting can begin to change when bystanders no longer walk past an anguished child without stopping to help. This may be the first time the child has been given the message that her feelings are legitimate and important, and she may remember this critical message later when she herself has a child.

Crying is a signal provided by nature. It is meant to disturb the parents

9. Crying is a signal provided by nature. It is meant to disturb the parents so that the child's needs will be met. It makes no sense that nature would have provided all children with a routinely used signal that serves no good purpose.

10. Parents who respond only to "good" behavior may believe they are training the child to behave "better." Yet they themselves feel most like cooperating with those who treat them with kindness. This is another example of

how children are seen as a different species, when in fact they are human beings who behave on the same principles as all other human beings. Like the rest of us, they respond best to kindness, patience, and understanding. Parents wondering why a child is "misbehaving" might stop and ask themselves this question: "Do I feel like cooperating when someone treats me well, or when someone treats me the way I have just treated my child?"

Siblings Arrive All at Once

A PARENT WROTE FOR ADVICE because she was having "power struggles" with her four-year-old daughter. While she shared many details about her little girl, her most helpful comment was that seven weeks earlier she had given birth to a baby boy.

A seven-week-old infant requires an enormous amount of time and attention. Siblings will inevitably receive less attention from their parents than they did before the baby arrived. No matter how well the parent prepares them for this change, it will be a major and sudden transition for them. One day Mother is still pregnant; the next day the baby has arrived.

If a baby could somehow appear gradually — if he could be present for one hour the first day, two hours the next day, and so on — there would be a gradual change in the amount of attention older children received from their parents. But babies arrive all at once, and siblings must do their best to adjust to this sudden lessening of their parents' time, energy, and attention.

It is our job as parents to understand this situation from the child's point of view. The better we are able to empathize with a sibling's inevitable feelings of disappointment and jealousy, the better we will be able to meet his need for attention. It can be a challenge when siblings require more attention than usual at the precise time that parents have less to give! Our own adjustment to the new baby has come suddenly too. It is for this reason that Dr. Elliott Barker, director of the Canadian Society for the Prevention of Cruelty to Children, recommends allowing at least three years between children so that the older child has a better chance of fulfilling his need for his parents' time and attention. According to Dr. Barker:

> *It requires an enormous amount of time and energy on the part of both parents to adequately nurture one child under the age of three. Spacing children is one important thing that parents can do to prevent the exhaustion that occurs when well-intentioned parents take on the very difficult task of trying to meet the emotional needs of closely spaced children.*[1]

While multiple births cannot be spaced, twins and triplets do not have the same challenges that an older sibling has, because they have never been an only child.

We might wish that an older child could understand the situation from our point of view and demand less attention from us while the baby is still small and helpless. But that is not the way things are, especially when children are closely spaced. It is simply not fair, realistic, or helpful to expect children to be able to postpone their urgent needs for our love and reassurance. It is our task to empathize with their needs. And our empathy for each child is precisely how they learn to have empathy for others — including their new brother or sister.

It is, as always, a matter of trust. We need to believe in our children. We need to understand that they are communicating their legitimate needs in the most mature way possible at that point in their development and circumstances. If we punish them for this communication, they cannot move on to more mature means of expressing their needs and feelings.

We need to find the love within our own hearts to empathize with a child who is faced with such a sudden and difficult adjustment. But how can a parent who is overextended after the birth of a baby find the energy to cope with an older child's feelings of rejection and jealousy?

Careful nutrition and adequate rest, both before and after the birth, can make a remarkable difference in our ability to cope with an older child's adjustment — and our own. Taking the time to prepare a child for a new sibling — through patient listening, full response to questions, sharing informative books, and spending time with babies in other families — can be helpful. But the most important factor will always be our capacity to love, respect, and trust each child.

Lonely Cages

All truth goes through three stages. First it is ridiculed. Then it is violently opposed. Finally, it is accepted as self-evident.

— Arthur Schopenhauer

T HIS STATEMENT, WRITTEN 200 years ago, has certainly passed the test of time. In the 16th century, Copernicus's writings, in which he claimed that the earth moves around the sun, were banned for decades, and Galileo's belief in that theory led to an Inquisition trial and house imprisonment. Today, of course, Copernicus's vision seems self-evident. Many of our other beliefs have taken the same progression, from ridicule to violent opposition and finally to acceptance as self-evident truth. Unfortunately, in recent times child-rearing practices seem to be moving in the opposite direction. In many areas, such as sleeping, feeding, and discipline, we started with a loving and trusting connection to our children and have moved toward an artificial, mistrustful, and distant approach, especially in the Western world.

For hundreds of thousands of years, the child's need to be close to parents during both day and night was a self-evident truth

Consider the now controversial issue of co-sleeping. For hundreds of thousands of years, the child's need to be close to parents during both day and night was a self-evident truth, the obvious way to respond to a child's legitimate need for closeness and comfort. Parents of long ago knew that their children deserved to have their company and their loving support in the darkness of the night as much as — or more than — they did in the light of day.

Babies slept next to their mothers, which fostered the bond between them and encouraged and facilitated breast-feeding. We now know that co-sleeping provides numerous benefits to babies:

- Family co-sleeping takes full advantage of the ease of breastfeeding, as a mother does not need to go to another room to get the child. She can easily feed her child without having to wake fully and can continue to get the rest she needs. Thus co-sleeping encourages mothers to extend breast-feeding and all of its numerous benefits for a longer time. As well, babies sleeping with their parents nurse three times as often during the night as do isolated babies, enjoying a more evenly spaced nutritional intake, as well as a somewhat larger volume of breast milk.[1]

- According to sleep researcher James McKenna, co-sleeping increases the chances that a parent can successfully intervene to help prevent a death, whether that is due to a physiological condition or to a physical accident. He reminds parents that "co-sleeping gives the parent the best opportunity to hear the baby in crisis and to respond." Gaps in breathing are normal during the early months of infancy, and it is likely that the mother's breathing provides important cues to her infant, reminding him to take a breath following exhalation. This can prevent a Sudden Infant Death Syndrome (SIDS or crib death) situation from developing. If this reminder system fails, the mother is nearby to help by arousing the infant. A breast-feeding mother and baby tend to have coordinated sleeping and dreaming cycles, making the mother keenly sensitive to her baby. If she is sleeping close by, she will awaken if her baby is having difficulty. If the baby is alone, this type of lifesaving intervention cannot take place. McKenna adds that "since protection from SIDS may be related to the frequency and duration of breastfeeding, and because babies breastfeed more when co-sleeping, this practice may help to protect some breastfeeding infants."[2]

• Any nighttime danger to a child is reduced if there is an adult close by. Cribs are dangerous and prevent parents from intervening quickly in emergencies. According to the U.S. Consumer Product Safety Commission, "More babies — about 40 to 50 each year — die in incidents involving cribs than with any other piece of nursery equipment."[3] Thousands more are injured seriously enough to require emergency treatment. Babies and children isolated in separate rooms have perished in fires, been sexually abused by overnight visitors, been abducted from their beds, been attacked by pets, or have died or been injured in various ways. Many, if not all of these tragedies might have been averted had the parent been present and aware of the baby's well-being throughout the night.

- Suffocation is often listed as a danger of family co-sleeping. However, this is a real danger in only two situations: when an infant is sleeping on a waterbed and is thus unable to push herself up when needed; or when a parent is too intoxicated by alcohol or drugs to attend to a child's needs. Obviously a child who is suffocating for any reason (such as a ribbon on sleepwear getting around her neck, vomiting during sleep, asthmatic attacks) is far more likely to rouse a parent who is sleeping nearby than one sleeping in a different room.

- Family co-sleeping is often misunderstood as an opportunity for parents to sexually abuse their children. In fact, parents who develop deep emotional bonds with their children by remaining close by and responsive at night, as well as during the day, are far less likely to turn to abusive behavior of any kind toward the children they love and cherish. Conversely, the fact that a child sleeps alone has never been adequate protection against a parent who intends sexual trespass and may even make it easier for one parent to keep such activity secret from the other. Cribs make babies even more vulnerable and unprotected.

- Shared sleep can further prevent child abuse by allowing all family members to obtain the rest they need, especially if the child is breast-feeding. The child does not have to suffer needlessly or cry to bring his mother, and the mother can nurse half-asleep. The entire family awakes refreshed, with no lingering resentment toward the baby for having disturbed their sleep the night before. An exhausted parent is far more likely to abuse a child than a well-rested mother or father who has enjoyed the presence of a happily resting child through the night.

- Crying is a natural signal that is meant to disturb parents to ensure that their baby receives the care she needs. Prolonged crying is stressful to all family members. The sooner the baby's needs are met, the more rest the baby and the entire family can have, and the more energy they will have for the next day. A mother sleeping next to her baby uses the instinctive response a new mother has to her baby's first whimper, thus preventing the need for the hard crying that is so stressful to the baby and the whole family.

- Studies of adults in coma show that the presence of another person in the room significantly improves heart rate, heart rhythm, and blood pressure. It seems reasonable to assume that infants and children derive similar health benefits from having others in the same room with them.

- A deeper sense of love and trust often develops between siblings who sleep near each other, lessening sibling rivalry during waking hours. Siblings who share the night as well as the day have a greater opportunity to build a deep and lasting relationship. Babies and children who are separated from other family members during the day, when parents are at work and siblings at school, can partially make up for these absences and reestablish important emotional bonds by spending time at night together. Of course, home businesses and unschooling can minimize separations and deepen family bonds during the day, just as co-sleeping does at night.

The parents of long ago (and of most Third World countries today) didn't weigh these benefits against any other approach; they simply followed their instinctive drive to love, protect, and nurture their children in the most natural ways.

Why have we moved in the opposite direction? Why do we not abandon cribs, where many babies have died and many more have been injured? When babies die in cribs, parents are never told to avoid them; we hear only pleas for safer products. But when a baby dies in a bed, it draws calls for an end to co-sleeping, with little attention paid to the actual cause of that death (usually the result of an intoxicated parent, a waterbed, or a gap between the mattress and the frame). Instead of calling for the end to such an age-old, beneficial and healthy arrangement, we should investigate the specifics of each situation, and educate parents about safety measures.

Cribs force babies to face the long night alone years before they are psychologically equipped to do so. Isolation teaches harmful messages of mistrust, forces "cooperation" through despair, and instills a deep sense of loneliness that no teddy bear can fulfill. Judging from the reports of adults in hypnotherapy, art therapy, and psychoanalysis, experiences of isolation from parents in infancy and childhood can be traumatic, with harmful repercussions on the adult personality. It seems reasonable to assume that there is not one baby in the world who would choose cold isolation over loving proximity if given the choice. Our babies' cries and screams should be more than sufficient to convince us of the emotional harm and moral wrongness of such separation. Why do we not hear what they try so hard to tell us?

A child who is cared for during the night as well as the day receives constant reassurance of love and support instead of having to cope with feelings of fear, anger, and abandonment night after night. Children who have felt safe at night with a loving parent close by, become adults who cope better with the inevitable stresses life brings. As John Holt put it so eloquently, having feelings of love and safety in early life, far from "spoiling" a child, is like "money in the bank:" it provides a fund of trust, self-esteem, and inner security that the child can draw on throughout life's challenges.[4]

Cribs seriously lessen the critical emotional bond between parent and child, and between siblings. Cribs keep working parents from spending their only available block of free time with their children. Cribs are lonely cages for babies who deserve to have their age-old needs met with love and respect. Cribs have no real benefits at all. Let's abolish them!

Ten Ways to Grow a Happy Child

> The first real choice a human baby must make is whether to trust or mistrust other humans. This basic trust-versus-mistrust stage is the first building block upon which all later love relationships are formed.　　　　　　　— Dr. Ken Magid[1]

1. Fall in love with your baby by having a positive birthing experience for baby, mother, and father.

2. Strengthen that love by breast-feeding your child until he or she no longer needs it.[2] Breast-feed your baby until he or she no longer needs it. Breast milk contains immune-system enhancers that help keep your baby healthy. Any other food, even sugar water, permanently destroys many of these important substances. A healthy baby is a joy!

3. Breast-feeding is also good for mothers. A nursing mother produces hormones that help her to be patient and loving, making parenting easier. As well, a breast-feeding mother and her infant share sleep cycles and dream in unison, so the mother is less likely to be awakened by her baby during dreams or deep sleep. A refreshed mother is a patient mother!

4. Keep your baby with you as much as possible. Separations and changing caretakers make it harder for your child to learn trust and to grow into a loving and trusting adult.

5. Share sleep with your baby. This makes nighttime parenting easier and can help prevent Sudden Infant Death Syndrome. Your child's need for your presence does not magically disappear at bedtime.

6. Respond quickly and compassionately to your baby's cries, both day and night. This reassures him that he is important to you. Picking up your baby will not "spoil" him. Carrying him increases brain cell connections. According to Dr. George Wootan:

> *The increased opportunity for parent-child bonding offered by breastfeeding is a widely known benefit of nursing, which brings up an interesting sidelight. A baby can have lots of brain cells, but they won't do any good unless they're interconnected. The nerve fibers that connect these cells are called dendrites. And what develops dendrites? You probably said breast milk ... right? Wrong! Touching develops dendrites. Holding, touching, and stroking a baby, as a mother naturally does while nursing ("you can prop a bottle but not a breast"), helps the child develop the way nature intended, both physically and emotionally*[3]

You can't love a baby too much!

You can't love a baby too much!

7. A close bond between mother and child, naturally achieved through breastfeeding, holding, and shared sleep, is the best prevention of child abuse.

8. Remember that punishment teaches violence, destroys self-esteem, creates anger, interferes with learning, and damages the relationship between parent and child. "People are not for hitting, and kids are people too!"[4]

9. Allow your child's sense of trust plenty of time to grow strong before having a new baby to claim your attention. A three- or four-year spacing between children reaps enormous emotional benefits for each child.[5]

10. "Bad behavior" is a sign that a child's basic needs have not been met. Remember to give your children undivided attention, eye contact, and touching, and try to see things from their point of view. The best gifts you can give your child are your time, patience, and understanding.

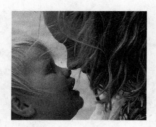

LIVING WITH CHILDREN

Ten Ways We Misunderstand Children

1. **We expect children to be able to do things before they are ready.** We ask an infant to keep quiet. We ask a two-year-old to sit still. We ask a four-year-old to clean his room. In all of these situations, we are being unrealistic. We are setting ourselves up for disappointment, and setting the child up for repeated failures to please us. Yet many parents ask their young children to do things that even an older child would find difficult. In short, we ask children to *stop acting their age.*

2. **We become angry when a child fails to meet our needs.** A child can only do what he can do. If a child cannot do something we ask, it is unfair to expect or demand more, and anger only makes things worse. A two-year-old can only act like a two-year-old, a five-year-old cannot act like a ten-year-old, and a ten-year-old cannot act like an adult! To expect more is unrealistic and unhelpful. There are limits to what a child can manage, and if we don't accept those limits, it can only result in frustration on both sides.

3. **We mistrust the child's motives.** If a child cannot meet our needs, we assume that he is being defiant. To determine the truth of the matter, we need to look closely at

53

the situation from the child's point of view. In reality, a "defiant" child may be ill, tired, hungry, in pain, responding to an emotional or physical hurt, or struggling with a hidden problem such as food allergy. Yet we overlook these possibilities while thinking the worst about the child's personality.

4. **We don't allow children to be children.** We forget what it was like to be a child and expect our children to act like adults instead of acting their age. A healthy child will have a short attention span, and be rambunctious, noisy, and emotionally expressive. All of these so-called problems are not problems at all, but are in fact normal attributes of a normal child. Rather, it is our society and our society's expectations of perfect behavior that are abnormal.

5. **We get it backwards.** We expect, and demand, that the child meet our needs — for quiet, for uninterrupted sleep, for obedience to our wishes, and on and on. Instead of accepting our parental role to meet the *child's* needs, we expect the child to care for *our* needs. We become so focused on our own unmet needs and frustrations that we forget this is a child, who has needs of her own that she cannot meet herself.

6. **We blame and criticize when a child makes a mistake.** Children have had little life experience, and they will inevitably make mistakes. Mistakes are a natural part of learning at any age, but instead of understanding and helping the child, we blame him, as though he should be able to learn everything perfectly the first time. To err is human; to err in childhood is human and unavoidable. Yet we react to each mistake, infraction of a rule, or so-called misbehavior with surprise and disappointment.

7. **We forget how deeply blame and criticism can hurt a child.** Many parents are coming to understand that physically hurting a child is wrong and harmful, yet many of us forget how painful angry words, insults, and blame are to a child, who can only believe that she is inadequate, incompetent, and unloved.

8. **We forget how healing loving actions can be.** We fall into vicious cycles of blame and misbehavior, instead of stopping to give the child love, reassurance, self-esteem, and security with hugs and kind words. As Mother Theresa wrote, "Kind words can be short and easy to speak, but their echoes are truly endless."

9. **We forget that our behavior provides the most potent lessons to the child.** It is truly not what we say, but what we do that the child takes to heart. A parent who hits a child for hitting, telling him that hitting is wrong, is in fact teaching that hitting is *right*, at least for those in power. It is the parent who responds to problems with peaceful solutions who is teaching a child how to be a peaceful adult. Problems and challenges present our best opportunities for teaching values, because children learn best by experiencing real-life situations.

10. **We see only the outward behavior, not the love and good intentions inside the child.** When a child's behavior disappoints us, we should, more than anything else we do, assume the best. We should assume that the child means well and is behaving as well as possible considering all the circumstances (both obvious and hidden from us) as well as her life experience. If we always assume the best about our child, the child will be free to *do* her best. If we give only love, love is all we will receive.

Ten Tips for Shopping with Children

1. **Remember that children have limits.** If you are shopping with children, be alert to their needs. Are they tired, hungry, overexcited by the noise and confusion, or simply in need of fresh air and exercise or a reassuring hug?

2. **Remember that children are naturally curious.** Children are curious; this is how they learn about the world around them. If they want to examine an attractive item, scolding should be avoided. Instead, help them to hold the item safely or let them know that it can be viewed but not touched. You might say, "This is breakable, so let's just look at it together." Even if you cannot purchase an item, it can be helpful to share the child's enthusiasm and interest in it.

3. **Shopping with infants.** Shopping with an infant will be far easier if you make the trip after he is rested and fed. Babies and small children can become dehydrated in the dry air of shopping malls, so be sure to take frequent nursing or juice breaks. Babies are almost always happier when carried. A sling or carrier you wear provides far more comfort and emotional security than a stroller or grocery cart. A small childproof toy can help a baby cope with your inevitably lessened attention, but remember to

stop as often as possible and take a moment for gentle words, eye contact, and hugs.

4. **Shopping with toddlers.** You can begin to include toddlers in shopping decisions. Asking the child questions such as "Which of these peaches looks better to you?" can turn a boring, frustrating experience into a pleasurable one for both you and your child. Children of all ages enjoy and appreciate being able to make some of the product choices themselves. It's a good idea to bring along juice, a favorite snack, and a well-loved picture book or a newly borrowed one from the library. Being surrounded by a crowd of adults can intimidate small children, especially when stores are busy. Use a backpack to bring a toddler up to a height where she is more contented. This can also prevent the common, frightening experience of losing a toddler in a crowd.

5. **Shopping with older children.** An older child can be a great help on a shopping trip if you approach it in a spirit of fun and appreciation. Clip pictures of food from the newspaper grocery ads and bring them along so the child can help to locate the item. Children who are mature enough to shop by themselves can help shorten the trip by finding items alone, returning periodically to put items into the cart.

6. **Avoid the crowds.** Shopping just before dinner, when stores are crowded and parents and children are tired and hungry, can be very stressful. Try shopping in the morning or early afternoon on weekdays, or have dinner early and shop during the quiet time between 6 and 7 p.m. When we avoid the stress of crowded stores and long

checkout lines, we have more energy and creativity for responding to our child's needs.

7. **The check-out lane can be a challenge.** Checkout lanes stocked with colorful, enticing gum and candy packages can be a real challenge, especially as you encounter them at the end of a shopping trip, when both you and your child are most fatigued and hungry. An easy alternative is to bring a favorite healthful snack from home: "That package looks pretty, but candy isn't very nutritious. Here's the oatmeal cookie and juice we brought." Shopping at stores that have "child-friendly" checkouts without candy can be well worth a longer drive. If there is no local store with such a checkout, you might suggest this feature to a store manager, promising to shop regularly if this option is made available.

8. **When you need to say "no."** The most important part of saying "no" is conveying to the child that you are on his side, even if you can't satisfy all desires immediately. It might help to say, "That is nice, isn't it? Take a good look and when we get home, we'll add it to your wish list." As the educator John Holt once said, "There is no reason why we cannot say 'No' to children in just as kind a way as we say 'Yes.'" And remember that smiles, hugs, and cuddles are all free!

> *The most important part of saying "no" is conveying to the child that you are on his side*

9. **If you reach your limit.** If you reach the limit of your patience and energy, try to show by example positive ways of handling anger and fatigue. You might say, "I'm starting to lose my patience. I think I need a break from shopping. Let's go outside for a few minutes so we can

both get refreshed." Even a few moments of fresh air away from the crowds can make a big difference for both parent and child. If you're doing your grocery shopping, there's no reason not to leave a half-filled cart for a short time. I often remind harried parents that "The store won't mind if you leave your cart here for a few minutes while you go outside with your child for some fresh air and a little exercise." They're always grateful for this suggestion. It's odd that we all think we need to watch our carts every minute — after all, we haven't paid for anything yet!

10. **If your children reach their limit.** If, after you've tried some of the above suggestions, your children have simply reached the end of their ability to handle any more errands, consider leaving. Shopping can wait; an exhausted, hungry, or overly excited child cannot.

Remember that all children behave as well as they are treated. A child who is regularly given our time, undivided attention, patience, and understanding will have more tolerance for a shopping trip — and any other challenging situation — than the child who must face stressful situations without this emotional support.

When a Child has a Tantrum

A s JOHN DONNE WROTE, "No man is an island;" we are always responding to the world around us, as well as to all that is happening within us. Yet it can be easy for us to

look at a child's behavior as though it is unrelated to anything else — as though the child is living in isolation from
the world around him. We must realize that a child's behavior is a response to the circumstances present at the time.
Those circumstances may be external — such as overstimu-
lation, stressful events, or sibling conflict — or they may be
internal — such as teething, food allergy, insufficient sleep,
or a developing illness.

We all know there are many causes of "misbehavior,"
yet it is surprisingly easy to see only the behavior, without
regard to what may have brought it about. For example, one
day when my son was two, we were about to enter our
house when he wandered off to explore a neighbor's yard.
This was frustrating for me, because I had numerous chores
I needed to do inside. I tried to convince him to leave, but
he was determined to remain there and continue his explo-
rations. The more frustrated I became, the more determined
he became, and we began to have a real power struggle.
Then I reflected for a moment and remembered that this
was a particularly stressful day for us all — we were moving
into a new house and had just arrived there after a long trip!
I am amazed now, as I recall the incident, that I could have
forgotten such a critical piece of information, but it is easy
to focus entirely on our child's behavior and our own frustration, even when there is a ready explanation. In fact, my
son was doing an understandable and intelligent thing:
becoming familiar with his new surroundings.

When a child has a tantrum, we may feel sorry for ourselves and puzzled about the causes, especially if we have
diligently met the child's needs in the past. Despite reassur-
ances from attachment parenting books and advisors, we

may easily begin to wonder whether the rest of the world isn't right — that children can become "spoiled" and that our child's behavior shows we have been wrong to trust him to grow to responsible adulthood without punishment and disciplinary measures.

At those times it can be helpful to stop thinking about all the reasons why our child shouldn't be behaving in this way — to stop thinking about all the love and attention we've given him over the years — and focus instead on the present. After all, the present moment is where each child lives. What has happened that day, that hour, the last few minutes? Just as I momentarily forgot that it was moving day, we can also forget such matters as a toy being broken, another child getting more attention, a meal with too much sugar, a noisy environment, a lengthy shopping trip, a visitor taking up our attention, a poor night's sleep, teething, a developing cold that hasn't shown itself yet, and so on.

We also need to consider the effect our own response is having — are we helping the situation by validating feelings ("You want to learn about all the new things here! Let's spend a few minutes now, and then come back soon."), or have we simply responded with our own frustration ("Come on! We have to go inside now! Right now!")?

In addition to looking at the circumstances just prior to a tantrum, we can also learn something by looking at the circumstances when the child is happy and relaxed. What has happened prior to *that* behavior? Has she enjoyed a relatively quiet day following a restful sleep? Have her parents recently solved a problem of their own? Have there been no trips and few telephone calls that day?

Has she had an especially nutritious meal? Has she just had plenty of one-on-one time with her parents?

It is all a matter of focus. We tend to focus on the entire history of our parenting ("I've been such a good mother. I've given him so much time, attention, and love. Why is he behaving like this?"). But this type of thinking is unrealistic. No child behaves perfectly at all times — neither does any adult. It is also unhelpful, because it doesn't lead us to solutions. If we can focus on the present circumstances — the knocked-over Lego building, the noise, the fatigue of shopping, the numerous phone calls that day, the teething — we are then able to answer the "why" question and move on to a helpful response of empathy and validation: "It's so hard for you when I have lots of phone calls, and now your sister knocked over your building! You must be feeling really frustrated!"

If we respond with anger, punishment, or rejection, it will only make things worse, as we give the child even more reasons to feel angry and frustrated, just when he is least able to handle it. The best approach is to express empathy while validating the child's feelings: "Oh, dear — the baby knocked over your beautiful Lego house again! How frustrating!" or "It must be hard for you to have to share me with your sister. You wish you could have me all to yourself right now!"

Giving children a time-out may appear to work as a short-term solution, but removing the child from the rest of the family can give an unintended and harmful message of conditional love: "We love you when you behave, but if you misbehave you're no longer welcome in our family."

When a child is having a tantrum, the key word is "helplessness." A tantrum develops when a child feels that he has no control over his circumstances; he wants things to be different, but he is helpless to bring about those changes. And helplessness brings fear — after all, he is at the mercy of other people's wishes. Helplessness also affects the child's self-esteem. When he feels powerless to change things, he may begin to believe that he is not capable of having, or does not deserve to have, his desires fulfilled.

In some ways it is a good sign when a child continues to insist that her needs be met. It means she trusts her parents to listen to her, she believes in herself, and she believes that she deserves to be heard and to have a say in the way her life unfolds. When a child is thwarted too often, she may stop asserting herself altogether.

> *A tantrum is a child's attempt to communicate the best way she can at the time.*

Unfortunately, such passive acceptance can be misinterpreted as a healthy response, when in fact the child has simply given up, while suppressing feelings of anger and frustration until she feels strong enough to resist — usually in adolescence. A tantrum is a child's attempt to communicate the best way she can at the time.

Always remember that a tantrum is a signal of helplessness and fear, even though it may give the opposite impression: that the child is trying to be more powerful than we are. Unfortunately, because few of us were given understanding words and validation of feelings in our own childhood, it can be easy — especially when we are feeling tired, upset, or powerless in our own life — to focus on the behavior rather than the feelings. After all, that is the example so many of us have had.

It can be especially difficult for empathic parents who lose their temper during stressful times, because we expect more of ourselves and of our children. We may be expecting too much of ourselves, considering our own upbringing and current stress level, and too much of our children, considering their age and lack of experience. It may be most helpful at those times to reflect that all parents do as well as they can, given all the circumstances of their life. The same is true for our children.

The Hidden Messages We Give Our Children

Newborn

What we say: "You can cry all you want; I'm not going to pick you up again!"

What we think: "This is breaking my heart, but all those experts can't be wrong."

What the child thinks: "They don't love me. They don't care about my suffering. Mommy is perfect, so there must be something wrong with me. I must not be worthy of anybody's love."

What we say 20 years later: "What on earth do you see in Tom? How can you let him treat you like that? Don't you know you deserve better than that?"

Infant

What we say: "No more nursing. You're too big for that now!"

What we think: "I'd like to continue, but I can't stand all this criticism from my relatives."

What the child thinks: "I've just lost the most important thing in my life: the long periods of cuddling and the food that felt best inside me. I must have done something terrible. I must be a terrible person."

What we say 20 years later: "Why are you drinking so much?"

Age Two

What we say: "You can't come into our bed anymore. You won't be lonely. Look, here's a nice big teddy bear to keep you company!"

What we think: "Grandma thinks there's something wrong with having you in our bedroom. I'm not sure what it is, but it's more important for us to please her than to please you. Anyway, this teddy bear should make you happy."

What the child thinks: "It isn't fair! They get to cuddle with a real person. They don't know me very well. They don't care about my feelings. Oh well, at least they gave me this bear."

What we say 20 years later: "I know you're upset that Tom broke off with you, but is that any reason to overcharge your credit card like this? Will all this stuff make you feel better that someone left you? When did you become so materialistic?"

Age Four

What we say: "You know you're not supposed to hit your brother! I'll give you a spanking you'll never forget!"

What we think: "There must be a better way to handle this, but it's what my dad did, so it must be right."

What the child thinks: "I was so upset with my brother I hit him. Now Dad is so upset with me for hitting, he's hitting me. I guess it's okay for adults to hit, but not for kids. I wonder what I should do when I get upset? Oh well, one of these days I'll be an adult myself."

What we say 20 years later: "A barroom brawl? Adults don't hit people just because they're upset. I never taught you to resort to violence!"

Age Six

What we say: "Well, this is a big day for you. Don't be afraid. Just do everything your teacher says."

What we think: "Please don't embarrass me by acting up at school!"

What the child thinks: "But I'm afraid! I'm not ready to leave them for so many hours a day! They must be getting tired of me. Maybe if I do what the teacher says, they'll like me better and let me stay home."

What we say 20 years later: "What?! Your friends talked you into taking drugs? Do you do what everybody else tells you to do? Don't you have a mind of your own?"

Age Eight

What we say: "Your teacher says you aren't paying attention in class. How will you ever learn anything important?"

What we think: "If my kid never amounts to anything, I'll feel like a failure."

What the child thinks: "I'm not interested in the things the teacher talks about, but I guess she knows best. The things that do interest me must not be important."

What we say 20 years later: "You're 28 years old and you still don't know what you want to do with your life? Aren't you interested in anything?!"

Age Ten

What we say: "You broke another dish? Oh, never mind. I'll wash them myself."

What we think: "I know I should be more patient with you, but at least this way the dishes will get done."

What the child thinks: "Boy, am I clumsy. I'd better not even try to help anymore."

What we say 20 years later: "You want that job but you won't even apply for it? You should have more faith in yourself!"

Age Twelve

What we say: "Go out and play with your friends — you'll have more fun with them than hanging around here all day."

What we think: "I know I should spend more time with you, but I've got so much to do. It's a good thing there are so many kids around here."

What the child thinks: "I want to do things with Mom and Dad, but they're always too busy. I guess my friends like me better."

What we say 20 years later: "You never call us or come to see us anymore. Don't you care about our feelings?"

Age Fourteen

What we say: "Please leave the room, dear. Your father and I have something personal to discuss."

What we think: "We have some secrets we'd rather you didn't know about."
What the child thinks: "I'm not really part of this family."

What we say 20 years later: "You're in prison?! Why didn't you tell us you were having problems? Don't you know there are no secrets in families? We tried so hard. Where did we go wrong?"

Ten Tips for Finding a Medical Professional for Your Child

The right to the best possible medical treatment is
a fundamental right, especially for children.
— UNESCO

1. Well before treatment is needed, help your child to prepare emotionally for medical procedures. Play "dentist," "doctor," or "hospital" and read relevant books about children having medical treatment. To help your child become familiar with medical instruments, find real instruments (such as a rubber pick and plastic dental mirror) or create "play" ones (for example, use a piece of fabric as a blood pressure cuff). Medical treatment can be frightening to a child, especially if there are too many new, strange, and frightening things to learn about all at once.
2. Find respectful, kind, and skilled caregivers now, and ask that your family be accepted as their patients. If there is an emergency, you won't have time to check recommendations. Ask someone whose opinions you trust (a friend,

another parent, a La Leche League leader, a midwife) to recommend professionals who genuinely like children and respect their needs. Alternative medicine offers other choices, such as naturopathic dentists and holistic pediatricians. Such personnel are often especially patient and kind with children, and it can be well worth the extra effort to find them if it helps you avoid traumatic medical experiences.

3.   Unless you have an emergency, always meet the staff before scheduling an appointment. Be aware that many adults, regardless of their profession, do not "get it." They don't understand that children deserve to be treated with dignity and respect. Don't assume that someone who went to dental, nursing, or medical school necessarily understands the critical importance of early childhood experiences. This essential topic was almost certainly not covered in their classes. (A pediatric dentist once criticized me for nursing my toddler, even though one of the many benefits of nursing is that it helps set the jaw properly, which prevents the need for braces later on.)

To find a professional who will work in close partnership with your child as well as you, always bring the child with you to see how the two interact. It is not enough to rely on a glowing recommendation. Another family may have had a good experience because of factors that do not apply to you or your child. The doctor may have had more personal rapport with the other family; he or she may have been in a better mood at the time; the child may have been older, more outgoing, or have had previous positive experiences with medical visits. The procedure may also have been different and not as difficult.

Also, be aware that no matter how cordial the staff may seem during a preliminary meeting, it is hazardous to assume that they will respect your child's needs and requests when they are busy with the medical procedures and following hospital protocol.

4. Medical professionals will often ask that you leave your child alone with them. The usual argument for parent-child separation is that it allows medical personnel to "better do their work." A helpful reply is that you *also* have work to do — providing critically important emotional support — and that with both of you doing your respective jobs, your child will receive the best possible care. Research clearly shows that anyone — child or adult — recuperates better and more quickly if given strong emotional support, and someone closely bonded to the child can best provide this. The "Charter of Rights for Children in Hospitals" includes recommendations that also apply to office visits.[1] Be polite but assertive ("I'll be staying with her" or "I'd prefer to stay, thank you"), and stay with your child as if they have given permission.

5. Be aware that children — like the elderly — often receive less pain medication than adults do. A child can experience great pain but feel powerless to ask for help. Stay on your child's side by validating his experience, and never hesitate to ask that immediate and sufficient pain relief be given to your child.

6. Ask for a *detailed*, step-by-step description of what will happen during the entire appointment. If the staff is reluctant to give you this information, go elsewhere. When my son needed dental surgery, I asked for and received a detailed description of the procedure.

Unfortunately, I was not told that they would take him forcefully from my arms and rush him into surgery, locking me out of the room and ignoring my protests!

7. Medical personnel can be intimidating and critical when their procedures are questioned. When a child needs medical treatment, the parent is naturally distracted and worried, making clear communication more difficult. For these reasons, it can be helpful to bring along an ally — a spouse, friend, or relative with similar views — to step in if you are having difficulty communicating your wishes and to show that your requests are not unique or odd. Your friend may also have creative solutions that you have not considered, such as holding the child on your lap during a dental appointment.

8. If the procedure is an elective one, remember that your legal consent is needed. If all else fails and your child's critical needs for support and comfort are being ignored, make it clear that you can and will withdraw permission. Ask to speak to the head nurse, department head, or hospital administrator. Don't be deceived by a nurse's claim that "There is no one higher," which I was once told. Again, having an ally present can be helpful if the situation requires a confrontation. Remember that *you owe far more to your child than to strangers*, regardless of their professional status.

> Be especially careful about making promises to your child that you may not be able to keep.

9. Be especially careful about making promises to your child that you may not be able to keep. For example, before promising to be present in the recovery room, be sure that this is possible and that all relevant personnel are

informed of this plan. Although I had permission from my son's doctor to be present when he awoke, the nurses on duty that day had not been informed. Broken promises endanger the trust between parent and child and should always be avoided.

10. Finally, send a letter after the procedure, letting the staff know what worked and what didn't work. This type of feedback is essential for effecting positive changes in our medical institutions. Try not to limit such letters to negative experiences. Applauding the efforts of staff members who were particularly supportive, specifying what they did and why it helped, can be the most useful feedback of all.

Even the most meticulous planning won't eliminate surprises arising from dental/medical procedures or policies. If something goes amiss, be prepared to validate your child's feelings of being abandoned or betrayed. Accept the anger and allow it to be expressed safely (provide pillows for pounding or art material for pictures about the experience), and accept and express your own anger and disappointment. Tell your child how you feel now, what you wish you had done at the time, and what the child deserved to have from you and from the doctor. Empathize with his feelings and reassure him that any mistakes were not deliberate on your part. Show with your words and actions that you are on his side, even though things went wrong. We can only do the best we can, learn from our mistakes, and plan to do better next time.

Natural Grandparenting

ABOUT 150 YEARS AGO, people began to recognize that the color of one's skin did not make someone less of a person, and laws were passed to protect people of color from abusive and unfair treatment. This bitter struggle has continued into the present, but most of us today understand that all people are entitled to the same rights and freedom in our society.

About 100 years ago, people began to understand that one's gender did not make someone less of a person, and laws were passed to protect women from abusive and unfair treatment. This too has been a bitter struggle, which has continued to the present, but most of us today understand that both men and women are entitled to the same rights and freedoms in our society.

About 25 years ago, people began to see that the age of one's body did not make someone less of a person, and that seniors were entitled to the same rights and freedoms as everyone else. Again, this struggle continues today.

In recent years we have finally begun to extend rights and freedoms to children. What does our struggle for children's rights mean for grandparents, who were raised in such different times? One outcome is that children are no longer seen as property, to be manipulated through threats and punishment to meet the needs of their parents and grandparents. We are beginning to see children as real persons with real feelings, to be treated with the same dignity and respect as everyone else.

Fifty years ago a grandchild was expected to show respect and courtesy to a grandparent, with little regard for the way the grandparent treated the child or for the child's true inner feelings towards the grandparent. Respect and courtesy are still highly valued today. The difference is that respect is beginning to be recognized as a two-way street, and the child's feelings are more often taken into account, along with the feelings of the older members of the family.

Grandparents are now in a position to receive genuine respect based on the child's love for them

There is good news and bad news here for grandparents. The bad news is that grandparents can no longer expect to be shown courtesy and respect simply by virtue of the fact that they reside on that particular branch of the family tree. Grandparents must make some effort to respect the child, to earn the child's respect, and to look at things from her point of view. But the good news is wonderful! Grandparents are now in a position to receive genuine respect based on the child's love for them, not merely an outward show of "manners" based on the child's fear of punishment.

Freedom is always contagious. More freedom for a grandchild means more freedom for the grandparent, who no longer needs to take the thankless role of the "feared elder," waiting passively for an empty show of respect. Grandma and Grandpa are now free to play the more active role of close, loving grandparents, with the emphasis on "grand!"

Today grandparents are called upon to listen carefully ("I can understand that you're feeling sad"), to judge fairly ("When you're four, you're entitled to act like a four-year-old"), to share feelings honestly but gently ("I'm so sorry, but I'm too tired to play right now"), to share their own experiences ("That reminds me of something that happened when I was four"), and to believe in the child's good intentions in all circumstances ("I guess you threw the pillow because you want to play with me, but is there something else we can do together?").

Because children today are recognized as real persons with real feelings, more effort is expected of both parents and grandparents. This may seem unfair; after all, they had to show respect to their own grandparents, regardless of how they were treated by them. But the gain for the elders is substantial. Grandparents of today are free to have real interactions with real persons, rather than formal, meaningless role-playing with a frightened child. Both grandparents and grandchildren have gained an exquisite freedom: to love and get to know someone real, and to be loved and known in return.

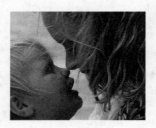

GUIDING
CHILDREN

The Parenting Golden Rule

"Treat all others as you would like to be treated yourself."

T HE GOLDEN RULE HAS PROVED its excellence as a moral guide since ancient times. Greek and Jewish thinkers, Confucius, Jesus, and other teachers of ethics all taught this rule, which is called "golden" to indicate its revered place as the ultimate rule of life. What better teaching can we use in our day-to-day approach to parenting? A variation of the Golden Rule for parents would be "Treat your child as you would like to be treated if you were in the same position."

It might be illuminating to consider this "Parenting Golden Rule" in relation to several common methods of discipline by placing a husband and wife in the same position as a child and parent.

1. Physical Punishment

The wife accidentally spills coffee on her husband's new jacket. He hits her.

Will the wife be more careful with his belongings in the future? Or might she have him arrested for spousal abuse?

79

2. Time-out

The husband starts to argue with a visiting friend. The wife tells him, "It's not nice to argue with your friend! I won't have this! Go sit in the bedroom for half an hour!"

Will the husband become less argumentative? Will the embarrassment of the situation set him straight? Will he feel like apologizing to his friend?

3. Consequences

The wife is out driving, forgets to fill the tank, and runs out of gas. She phones her husband to ask him to take his car to buy some gas and bring it to her. He refuses, explaining that she has to learn from "logical consequences" to be more responsible.

The next time the tank is low, will the wife remember to get it filled? Or will she be too preoccupied with fantasies of divorce to think about less important matters like car maintenance?

4. Counting

The wife reminds her husband, who is reading the newspaper after dinner, that it's his turn to do the dishes. He murmurs, "Mm hmm," and keeps on reading. The wife says, firmly, "You have to do the dishes now! Ten, nine, eight, seven ..."

Will the husband feel like cooperating with his wife? Or will he conclude that he's married a lunatic? And would he feel the least bit loved?

All of these disciplinary methods look ridiculous when viewed in this way. But at some point our society decided that children and adults respond to others according to different principles of behavior. This has been a harmful mistake. We have been asking the wrong question. We have asked, "Which set of rules works for children, and which set works for adults?" The reality is, happily, far simpler: all humans behave as well as they are treated. The only "method" that makes sense in a humane relationship with a fellow human being — whether a child or an adult — is unconditional love.

Parents wanting to help their children grow to be loving and responsible adults can do no better than to remember the Parenting Golden Rule: *"Treat your child as you would like to be treated if you were in the same position."* It's simple, straightforward, and effective. And we don't need to spend any time finding out what age someone is before consulting this rule. One size fits all.

The "Magic Words" Must be Spoken from the Heart

IN A LETTER TO THE EDITOR of an Oregon newspaper, the writer expressed a common complaint: several children had neglected to say "thank you" for the Halloween treats she had given them. She went on to say that the words themselves are the most important consideration and that parents should resort to force, if necessary, to extract them.

It is natural to feel hurt when it seems our kindness is being taken for granted. But maybe we should look a little more deeply. There are two entirely different reasons why a child would say "Thank you." One child may thank us because she is genuinely appreciative of our kindness, and has heard many expressions of gratitude within her own family — especially gratitude expressed to her.

Another child may say "Thank you," but may be mouthing empty words out of fear of punishment. Behavior based on fear, with little understanding of the reason for the ritual, is not only meaningless, but is also futile, as it fails to accomplish what we are seeking.

With threats of punishment, we may force a child to say "thank you," but we cannot force the genuine courtesy that we want. Real kindness grows within a child when he is treated kindly. It cannot be forced into his heart by forcing words into his mouth. Where is the joy in hearing "the magic words" spoken submissively by a frightened child? All words lose their magic if they are not truly spoken from the heart.

The educator John Holt once described a "real" thank-you that he received spontaneously from a young friend as a "lovely little present in words, full of pleasure, affection, and gratitude." He went on to say:

> As far as I can remember, this was the first time she had ever said "thank you" to me .... This little person has never been told to say "thank you." So why did she say it to me, if no one has told her to? How did she learn it? Because we adults always say "thank you" to her, and because she hears us saying it to one another. By keen observation she has picked it up that when

people do something nice for each other, it is a little gift of love, and the one receiving the gift gives a little gift back. Since she wants to do what we do, she did the same thing. In time, it will become as natural as breathing.

How different from another kind of scene, which I have witnessed many times: A child gazes on his gift, lost in pleasure, excitement and curiosity, when an adult voice says, often in a scolding or angry tone, "What do you say?" The child is snatched out of his world of awe and pleasure and is suddenly made to feel guilty and ashamed. He hears what he understands very well as a threat — if he doesn't say "thank you," something bad will happen to him. So, all pleasure gone, possibly even hating the present that has put him in this painful situation, he grudgingly and sullenly says "thank you."[1]

At Halloween, children also go to some effort, carefully selecting their new identity, getting dressed up, and walking for an hour or more. How many of us bother to say "Thank you for showing me your costume"? This is more than a question of fairness — it is the best teaching "method," because genuine courtesy comes most of all through imitation. Children learn to treat others with kindness by observing the adults around them doing kind things, and by hearing explanations, respectfully given, of the reasons for the behaviors we prefer.

Instead of complaining about rudeness in children, we should remember that children behave as well as they are treated and as well as they see us treating each other.

The Trouble with Rewards

A RECENT ARTICLE IN A PARENTS' magazine recommended using a "reward jar" for motivating children. The jar is filled with small toys or other rewards, to be given out when children complete certain specified tasks or change their behavior at the parent's request.

Parents who use rewards are motivated to find a less punitive method of helping their children to learn important things. It is "less punitive" rather than "non-punitive," however, because inherent in a reward system, whether voiced or not, is the possibility of failure — both failure to obtain the reward and failure to please the parent. Inevitably, the possibility of failure brings fear of failure.

Rewards, though on the surface so much more appealing than punishments, have some built-in risks and problems. The biggest problem is the hidden message that if there were no reward, the child would not want to perform the task in question. It can even be said that not being rewarded *is* a punishment.

When we offer rewards, children may receive these messages:

- The message that they are not able to recognize and appreciate on their own what is important to learn in life, and that they should learn only what others reward them for. They may then begin to disregard or question their own personal preferences and enthusiasms.

- The message that they can't trust their own judgments, that they should always seek an "expert" opinion before proceeding with a project, and that it is unwise to rely on their own perceptions and intuitions about the world around them. They may then begin to distrust their own choices and decisions.

- The message that the specific task being rewarded must be difficult or unpleasant, otherwise why has someone taken the trouble to set up a reward system? No one ever had to offer a reward to get a child to eat ice cream!

In addition to these unintended messages, there can also be some harmful results:

- If the parent takes an authoritarian role and determines how a child's difficulties should be resolved, the child loses the golden opportunity to practice problem-solving, and the family misses potentially better solutions the child may have invented if given the chance to do so.

- Extrinsic rewards take the child's attention away from intrinsic ones. The child may never understand the real reasons for doing something and may never appreciate the inherent rewards that a task will provide. For example, a child who reads a book in order to receive a sticker from the librarian may miss the point that reading is enjoyable all on its own.

In this sense, the child is being given less than a true picture of the world.

- Most importantly, the child's real needs may be missed and remain unmet, only to surface later. All of a child's behavior can be viewed as an outward manifestation of a legitimate inner need. Until that underlying need is dealt with fully, only superficial changes can take place. These underlying needs cannot be met through artificial, arbitrary rewards. A child's reluctance to go to bed may be a message about loneliness, rejection, or an impending illness, but that need will never be recognized if the problem is obscured by rewards. Instead he may receive the unintended message that his parents don't care about his feelings and needs, but merely want him to conform to their needs.

My own preference, when helping a child to learn a new task, is to stay focused on intrinsic rewards. All external rewards — whether tokens, school grades, gifts, or deliberate, manipulative praise — are arbitrary; that is, they bear no direct relationship to the matter at hand. Punishment has the same built-in problem. For example, if you are helping a child learn the importance of keeping her room orderly and clean, staying focused on the actual issue means helping the child to appreciate the *inherent* rewards: it's easier to find wanted items, she will avoid health problems (especially if she has allergies), there will be fewer broken toys or other kinds of damage, and most of us think more clearly and accomplish more in an orderly environment.

These kinds of explanations, if shared respectfully, will make more sense to the child than any external reward and will also show you trust her own abilities and motivations. This approach also has the benefit of helping the parent to determine priorities. If you can't explain the reason for doing something, maybe it isn't worth the effort of helping the child to do it! When you discuss tasks with your child, you may end up learning the most about priorities. To the child, keeping a room spotless at all times may be less important in the grand scheme of things than having time to play in an unhurried way with a parent or sibling.

Using a focused approach with an emphasis on intrinsic rewards also frees you to offer your child practical tips and actual help. You and your child remain on the same side, so you can both contribute ideas to make certain projects easier. When external rewards or punishments are used, you are more likely to feel that your child must perform the task alone.

When my son was young, I was fortunate to find books by John Holt and others that clarified the importance of focusing on intrinsic values. I began to believe that children could appreciate the benefits of such things as an orderly room, and I helped my son to identify the inherent rewards that orderliness brings. He felt free to ask for my advice and help, and I felt free to help him whenever necessary. Over time he learned that every effort to clean a room — or to carry out any other meaningful activity — brought its own rewards. He learned that such rewards are automatic and immediate. He is now 20, and his housekeeping skills and habits are far better than my own. I am still working on this area of my life, in part because of the stressful feelings that became associated with cleaning when I was young.

A good rule of thumb in parenting — or in any other relationship — is that anything that keeps us on the same side as our child is more respectful and consequently will be more successful than anything that sets up a hierarchy and puts a cold distance between us, such as parent-set standards and extrinsic rewards for specific behaviors.

By staying on the same side, we express trust in our child's ability to appreciate intrinsic rewards and to grow to be an adult who can think for himself, set his own standards and priorities, and iden-tify whatever inherent rewards are available through his own efforts. As my friend and colleague Mary Van Doren once noted, "Raising children with an emphasis on intrinsic rewards is not a technique, a method or a trick to get them to do what the parent wants them to by subtler means, but a way of life, a way of living with children with real respect for their intelligence and for their being."[1]

> *anything that keeps us on the same side as our child will be more successful*

The critical question is: What is it that we want? If we simply want a clean room, it may come about at an earlier age if we use rewards and punishments — but there may be unintended results: fears and unfortunate associations instilled in the child, damage to the parent-child bond, and the hidden message that the child cannot be trusted to learn without external motivators. The use of external rewards is a type of control, a method of manipulating our children to follow our agenda. All methods that rely on controlling the child have a price, paid by the child, the parent, and the relationship. Damage to self-esteem and self-knowledge is the highest price.

If we want more than the clean room — if we want the child to learn to appreciate intrinsic rewards, to have faith in his own judgment, to believe in his own ability to determine what is truly worth doing without seeking an authority fig-ure — it may take years longer, but it will be worth our extra effort and patience.

Parents who have taken the longer route of trusting and helping the child to gain self-motivation through a sen-sible appraisal of inherent rewards and values find that there are intrinsic benefits for them as well. It is far more reward-ing for a parent to raise a child who is independent, self-confident, realistic, and self-motivating, than it is to see an orderly bedroom at age six! If we use trust, patience, and gentle explanations instead of rewards or punishments, chil-dren are free to own their learning and personal growth. The less authoritarian we can be, while not relinquishing our role as our child's wise yet gentle guide, the more significant and lasting will be the learning that takes place.

Praising our Children:
Manipulation or Celebration?

IN RECENT YEARS, SEVERAL MENTAL HEALTH professionals have recommended that parents abstain from praise as well as criticism. They see praise as a form of parental manipulation of the child's behavior — more subtle than blame and criticism, but harmful nonetheless. I have cer-tainly seen parents using praise in this way. But I have also seen them use it in a way that I consider normal and healthy.

After much thought and discussion with colleagues, I have come to believe that avoiding all praise goes too far. While we should refrain from artificial, manipulative praise, there does exist a form of praise that springs from the heart in a joyful way and gives our children what they most need: our genuine loving support.

By "artificial praise" I mean words that are used deliberately to reinforce a specific behavior that leads toward a goal of the parent, and not necessarily of the child. Examples of manipulative praise include:

- "Tell Grandma thank-you. Good girl!"
- "Be a good boy and give your sister the toy ... good for you!"

By "genuine praise" I mean loving words that arise spontaneously and warmly from the parent's heart, without any thought of manipulation of the child's behavior. Examples of genuine praise include:

- "Wow! What a beautiful card you made for me! Thank you!"
- "Oh, you swept the floor! What a nice surprise!"

The key difference between these two kinds of praise is our intention. Are we simply expressing feelings of delight in the present moment, or do we intend to direct the child's future behavior by carefully giving or withholding our approval? Obviously if we mete out love and approval to our children when they are "good," and withhold it when they are "bad," we are taking serious liberties with our power over them. We are also giving the same harmful message that all punishment gives: the child is loved conditionally, only when he or she meets with our approval. It is every parent's responsibility to avoid this kind of manipulation.

However, if, as we try to avoid this, we are afraid to voice any positive statements at all, and withhold our true selves, we are missing the chance to share a genuine relationship with our child. In a sense, we are no longer fully present for the child. We may be giving up some of the most joyous moments in any relationship: the spontaneous words and gestures that celebrate the love and joy between us.

It Shouldn't Hurt to be a Child[1]

The birch is used only out of bad temper and weakness, for the birch is a servile punishment which degrades the soul even when it corrects, if indeed it corrects, for its usual effect is to harden.

— Saint John Baptiste de La Salle in
"On the Conduct of Christian Schools" (1570)

IN NORWAY AND SWEDEN it is illegal for a parent, teacher, or anyone else to spank a child. In some states and provinces of North America it is illegal for a teacher to spank, but in all parts of the continent, physical punishment by a parent, as long as it is not severe, is still seen by many as necessary discipline and condoned, or even encouraged.

For the past several years, however, many psychiatrists, sociological researchers, and parents have recommended that we ban the physical punishment of children. The most important reason, according to Dr. Peter Newell, coordinator of the organization End Punishment of Children

(EPOCH), is that "all people have the right to protection of their physical integrity, and children are people too."[2]

There are many other reasons to end spanking and other physical punishments.

- Hitting children teaches them to become hitters themselves. Extensive research data supports a direct correlation between corporal punishment in childhood and aggressive or violent behavior in the teenage and adult years. Virtually all dangerous criminals were regularly threatened and punished in childhood. It is nature's plan that children learn attitudes and behaviors through observation and imitation of their parents' actions, for good or ill, and physical punishment gives the message that hitting is an appropriate way to express feelings and to solve problems. If a child does not observe a parent solving problems in a creative and humane way, it can be difficult for him to learn to do this himself. As a result, unskilled parenting often continues into the next generation. It is the responsibility of parents to set an example of empathy and wisdom.

> *Virtually all dangerous criminals were regularly threatened and punished in childhood.*

- Punishment distracts the child from learning how to resolve conflict in an effective and humane way. A punished child becomes preoccupied with feelings of anger and fantasies of revenge and is thus deprived of the opportunity to learn more effective methods of solving the problem at hand or how to handle or prevent similar situations in the future. There is no specific information in a spanking, and any verbal direction — constructive or not — that is given at the time cannot be heard by a frightened, angry, and resentful child. The most timely opportunity for the child to learn something important has been lost.

- "Spare the rod and spoil the child," though much quoted, is in fact a misinterpretation of Biblical teaching. While the "rod" is mentioned many times in the Bible, it is only in the Book of Proverbs that this word is used in connection with parenting. In fact, King Solomon's harsh methods of discipline led his own son, Rehoboam, to become a tyrannical and oppressive dictator who narrowly escaped being stoned to death for his cruelty. In the Bible there is no support for harsh discipline outside of Solomon's Proverbs. Jesus saw children as being close to God and urged love, never punishment.[3] Love is defined in the Bible as being patient and kind [4]; hitting a child is neither patient nor kind.

- Punishment interferes with the bond between parent and child, as it is not human nature to feel loving toward someone who hurts us. The true spirit of cooperation that every parent desires can arise only through a strong bond based on mutual feelings of love and respect. Punishment, even when it appears to work, can produce only superficially good behavior based on fear. This good behavior will endure only until the child is old enough to resist. In contrast, cooperation based on respect will last permanently, bringing many years of mutual happiness as the child and parent grow older.

- Punishment does not accomplish the intended goal. It produces feelings of anger, resentment, and low self-esteem, not the genuine willing cooperation the parent seeks. Adults would also cooperate with someone who threatened or hit them, but they would do so only through fear, and only if the other person held more power. Genuine cooperation comes from the heart. The only cooperation worth having is that which is given freely by a child, not because he has been frightened into obedience, but because he feels loved, respected, and understood, and consequently wants to treat his parents with love and respect in return.

- Many parents never learned in their own childhood that there are positive ways of relating to children. When punishment does not accomplish the desired goals, and if the parent is unaware of alternative methods, punishment can escalate to more frequent and dangerous actions against the child. Sometimes parents justify spanking by saying they do it only when they are "calm." Although I wish no parent ever hit a child, I would prefer to hear that they spank only when they are angry; at least that would make some logical sense to the child and be consistent with what he is learning about human nature. If a parent is indeed "calm," then he should be able to think clearly enough to discover more creative and positive ways to resolve a problem.

- If the child cannot safely express anger and frustration, these feelings become stored inside. Anger that has been accumulating for many years can come as a shock to parents whose child now feels strong enough to express this rage, but angry teenagers do not fall from the sky. Punishment may appear to produce "good behavior" in the early years, but always at a high price, paid by parents and by society as a whole, as the child enters adolescence and early adulthood.

- All punishment is emotionally dangerous and mind-warping. Associating "love" with the deliberate infliction of pain is deeply confusing to a child, because children know in their hearts that love and pain are inconsistent. Spanking on the buttocks, an erogenous zone in childhood, can create in the child's mind an association between pain and sexual pleasure and lead to difficulties in adulthood. "Spanking wanted" ads in alternative newspapers attest to the sad consequences of this confusion of pain and pleasure.[5] If a child receives little parental attention except when being punished, the concepts of pain and pleasure become further entangled in the child's mind. A child in this situation will have little self-esteem, believing he deserves nothing better.

- Even "moderate" spanking can be physically dangerous. Blows to the lower end of the spinal column send shock waves along the length of the spine and may injure the child. The prevalence of lower back pain among adults in our society may well have its origins in childhood punishment. Some children have become paralyzed due to nerve damage caused by spanking, and some have died after mild paddlings because of undiagnosed medical complications.

- Physical punishment gives the dangerous and unfair message that "might makes right," that it is permissible to hurt other people, provided they are smaller and less powerful than you are. The child concludes that it is permissible to mistreat younger or smaller children, and when he becomes an adult, he may feel little compassion for those less fortunate than he is, while fearing those who are more powerful. This will hinder the establishment of meaningful relationships so essential to an emotionally fulfilling life.

- Punishment gives the child a message of rejection. The unbearable pain of being rejected by those who are so important to the child's very survival will require him to deny his true feelings. As it is too painful to believe that a loved parent is deliberately hurting him, the child instead begins to believe that punishment is appropriate and proper behavior for a parent, that a child misbehaves because he is "bad," and that "bad" children deserve to be hurt. It is in this way that misconceptions about children's behavior — and about the most helpful ways to respond to that behavior — continue through the generations.

- In many cases of so-called "bad behavior," the child is simply responding in the only way he can, given his age and experience, to the neglect of basic needs. It is surely wrong and unfair to punish a child for responding in a natural way to having important needs neglected. For this reason, punishment is not only ineffective in the long run, but is also clearly unjust.

It may be helpful to consider the most common reasons a child "misbehaves:"[6]

1. **The child is trying to fulfill a legitimate need that has been ignored too long.** She may be hungry, thirsty, overtired, or may simply need a reassuring hug or some undistracted respectful listening. Such needs can be met easily if the child has not had to wait too long (indeed most children are surprisingly patient), but if they are continually postponed, the result can be a lengthy conflict, with tantrums, crying, hitting, and other kinds of misbehavior. The proverb "A stitch in time saves nine" is most apt in parenting.

2. **The child lacks information.** An infant reaches for a hot object because she does not yet know about such hazards; a toddler "takes" an item in a store because she is simply too young to understand about stealing; a child runs into a street because she doesn't fully understand the dangers. If a child misbehaves due to a lack of information, it is our responsibility to provide the information. It is not the child's responsibility to know something she does not know. It is unfair and ineffective to punish a child because she lacked information, and a punished child will be too distracted by feelings of anger or resentment and fantasies of revenge to learn the lesson intended. In this way, punishment diverts the child's attention from the matter at hand and interferes with learning — at precisely the best time for this learning to take place.

3. **The child is emotionally upset or physically distressed.** He may be frightened, angry, confused, jealous, disappointed, or he may have other intense feelings because of whatever happened just prior to the misbehavior. He may

be "misbehaving" due to more subtle causes, such as the discomfort of an impending illness or the high histamine levels associated with allergy. It is not really so difficult to understand the reasons for a child's (or an adult's) behavior if we simply *put ourselves in their place*. Children are not an alien species; just like adults, they all behave as well as they are treated.

If we try to change a child's behavior without attending to these natural, universal, and understandable feelings and needs, we do not help the child, because the underlying problem has not been dealt with. Simply forcing a child, by means of our greater size and power, to meet *our* needs does not resolve the issues that led to the behavior. The unwanted behavior — or another kind of misbehavior — will recur until the child's legitimate needs are met, her feelings are understood and accepted, and she feels truly loved and secure.

It is inevitable that the child's needs will sometimes conflict with our own, but this is not the child's fault any more than it is the fault of one adult when the needs of two adults conflict. The difference is that parents are in a position of superior power, which they can — but should not — misuse.

punishment and misbehavior can quickly escalate into a vicious cycle

It is wrong and unfair for the strong to overcome the weak by force. Indeed, any negativity or force in conflict resolution simply creates more conflict. Because of this, punishment and misbehavior can quickly escalate into a vicious cycle, with parent and child locked in a struggle for power. The parent, having more power by virtue of his size, parental role, and one-sided laws that protect adults — but not children — from physical aggression, can always win such a struggle, at least until the child reaches the teenage years and is physically strong enough to rebel.

As children learn most clearly by example, true loving guidance consists of patience, trust, acceptance, and understanding shown to the child by the parents. Kind parents who treat their children with respect, understanding, and patient explanations find that this "method" continues to work — through infancy, toddlerhood, childhood, the teenage years, and beyond into adulthood. When the parent in later years is in need of care, the child will then happily return the love and assistance he was given in childhood.

As Canadian psychiatrist Dr. Elliott Barker wrote, "Kids who have their needs met early by loving parents ... are subjected totally and thoroughly to the most severe form of 'discipline' conceivable: they don't do what you don't want them to do because they love you so much!"[7]

"I Was Spanked and I'm Fine!"

WE HEAR IT ALL THE TIME when spanking is mentioned. Someone steps forward and says something like, "Well, I don't see what all the fuss is about. I was spanked, and I'm fine. We all know that spanking is sometimes necessary for solving problems with kids. And since it's both necessary and harmless, it should be allowed and even encouraged."

This seems to be an airtight case and a perfectly logical justification of spanking as part of the necessary discipline of children. But is it really so logical? Is spanking necessary? And is it as harmless as so many believe it to be? Let's examine the argument.

- "I was spanked." (Fact)
- "I'm fine." (Opinion)
- "Sometimes spanking is necessary for solving problems with kids." (False assumption)
- "Since it is both necessary and harmless, it should be allowed and even encouraged." (Invalid conclusion)

Now let's consider a similar argument that seems to justify smoking.

- "The comedian George Burns smoked all his life from his teenage years on." (Fact)
- "He was in reasonably good health all his life and lived to be 100." (Fact)
- "Sometimes smoking is necessary for coping with life's problems." (False assumption)
- "Since smoking is harmless and sometimes necessary, it should be allowed and even encouraged." (Invalid conclusion)

This comparison makes it clear that the spanking argument, like the one on smoking, is based on false assumptions and leads to invalid conclusions. Some children, like some smokers, are less affected than others because of a natural emotional resiliency, just as George Burns must have had physical resilience.

Some children, like some smokers, are less harmed than others because of mitigating factors, such as the presence of other adults who treat them with love and care. To the extent that a spanked child is really "fine," it is *in spite of*, not *because of*, the punishments they have received. George Burns must have had mitigating factors too. Perhaps his strict regimen of daily exercise helped him to fare better than other smokers, or perhaps he inherited a strong constitution. Research shows that laughter can be an important healer and that many professional comedians live long lives.

For many reasons, George Burns was one of the survivors among frequent smokers. And for many reasons there are also "survivors" of spanking. But we can never know just how much happier and more fulfilled they might have been had they been gently guided instead of being punished — anymore than we can know just how much healthier George Burns might have been had he never smoked a cigarette or a cigar. Would he have lived even longer, entertaining more people and writing more delightful books? Would he have brought joy, laughter, charm, and wisdom to yet another generation?

spanking is not only harmful; it is also entirely unnecessary

Like smoking, spanking is not only harmful; it is also entirely unnecessary because there are far more effective and emotionally healthy alternatives. These alternatives work in the long term — which spanking does not — because they establish a pattern of good behavior that is motivated by the simple, genuine desire to reciprocate love.

Behavior that is based on fear can last only until the child is old enough not to fear defying the parent. Punishment builds anger and resentment within the child that will inevitably be expressed at a future time. In contrast, behavior based on mutual love and trust will last through all the years of a child's life, and through the entire length of the parent-child relationship. There is nothing more rewarding for parents than the enduring, loving, and close tie with their children over many years.

Given all of this, let us revise the spanking argument:

- I was spanked.
- I'm fine, but I wish I were happier, more productive, and better able to love and trust others.
- Since spanking is both unnecessary and harmful, it should never be allowed. Our government, like those in many European nations, should actively and strongly discourage it.

Spanking, like all other forms of punishment such as time-out and so-called logical consequences, can only bring about temporary and superficially "good" behavior based on threats and fear. Spanking is unnecessary, harmful, disrespectful, and unfair. Gentle, loving, and respectful guidance is the only truly effective way to help a child to grow and develop to his full potential as a loving and trusting adult.

The Dangers of Holding Therapy

HOLDING THERAPY IS A PRACTICE that was first described and recommended in the book *Holding Time*, by Martha Welch.[1] In this practice, a therapist or parent holds a child until he stops resisting or until a fixed time period has elapsed. Sometimes the child is not released until there is eye contact. Although this technique was initially intended for autistic adults, it has also been used for autistic children, teenagers, younger children with "attachment disorders," and infants with "residual birth trauma."

Proponents of this practice defend it as being "for the child's own good," the same justification that many use for spanking and other punishments. Because it is labeled "therapy," it can be difficult to regulate professionals' use of this practice or to help parents recognize its dangers.

I consider holding therapy to be completely at odds with compassionate parenting, which is above all a relationship based on mutual trust. It can be immensely difficult for a child to regain full, genuine trust after being forcibly held — regardless of the parent's good intentions or the resulting surface behavior.

It is human nature to resent and resist the use of force. If a parent uses forced holding, it will inevitably engender strong feelings of fear, confusion, helplessness, anger, and betrayal as the child's natural attempts to break free are disregarded by those he has come to love and trust. When held by force, the child finally understands that freedom comes only by giving in to outside control — a dangerous lesson for a young child. His will can be broken, but that is not what I would call psychological health.

Holding therapy is believed by some to bring about breakthroughs in teenagers who have become repressed, enabling them to express anger — but at a great cost in lost trust in the person performing the forced holding. And even apparent "breakthroughs" can be deceptive. Children who have had this "therapy" report that they simply did whatever was necessary to end the session — feigning smiles and cooperation, while they felt angry, embarrassed, and frustrated inside. In this way, they are being taught that outward appearances are what matter, not inner feelings, and this can be the basis of future antisocial behavior. As with spanking and all other forms of punishment, the child may appear to comply while his deeper feelings are submerged until they can be more freely expressed. Further, where force is used, the authenticity of any "success" is forever in doubt. When a child cannot say "no," what does his "yes" really mean? Psychopathic individuals often learn to feign appropriate behavior that they do not truly feel inside. In contrast, emotionally healthy people express their true and deep feelings. Thus holding therapy can be seen as creating the opposite of psychological health.

the best alternative is prevention through meeting the child's legitimate needs

There is always a risk factor when force is used on a child, and it is never justified unless the child's life or health are immediately endangered and there is no better alternative. There *are* alternatives, many of them, to nearly all parental acts of forced submission. For the unhappy or out-of-control child, the best alternative is prevention through meeting the child's legitimate needs (giving her your undivided attention, making sure she has enough food and sleep, discovering and treating hidden allergies, relieving family-related stress factors, etc.). Where the use of force is unavoidable (when your child runs into the street, for example), it should be kept to the barest minimum possible and should be followed by gentle explanations and apologies.

I believe that forced holding where there is no immediate danger should be challenged on humanitarian grounds. And far from having health benefits, as proponents claim, it may also pose a serious psychological risk:

> *One of the most important advances in our under-standing of health and disease in the past few decades ... has been identifying the prototype of pathogenic [disease-creating] situations — being trapped in adverse or threatening circumstances and being unable to either fight or flee. When we can only passively submit, our health tends to deteriorate."*[3]

On the other hand, being in a position to take the initiative is health enhancing.

There is yet another compelling reason to challenge this procedure. How can we justify forced holding in a society where children are cautioned — for good reason — to say "no" to unwanted touch? Whether it is done by a parent, a therapist, or a stranger, physically overpowering a helpless child is wrong. Justifying it by calling it "love" or "therapy" is a violation of the child's trust and understanding of life as he has come to know it. Like all other forms of forced compliance, forced holding associates love and submission.

Gentle, empathic approaches are far less stressful for all concerned than forced holding; they are more effective for the long term and more respectful of the child, who deserves our love and compassion. It is sad that something as lovely as having a child in our arms — when the desire is mutual — has been perverted into such a heartless practice.

Ten Alternatives to Punishment

MANY PARENTS HAVE COME to recognize the harmful effects of physical punishment. They have learned that slapping, hitting, and spanking teach violence, destroy the child's self-esteem, create anger, interfere with learning, and damage the relationship between parent and child.

But knowing what *not* to do is only the first step. Parents who want to avoid punishment wonder what they should do instead. Unfortunately, most parenting books and articles recommend "alternatives" that, on closer inspection, turn out to be merely alternative types of punishment. These include so-called logical consequences, time-out, and denial of privileges.

All of these methods have much in common with physical punishment, and all give the same messages: that the parent has no interest in the underlying unmet needs that led to the behavior, and that the parent is willing to take advantage of his greater size and his power over the child. Above all, they tell the child that the people he has come to love and trust wish to cause him pain. This is a "crazy-making" message because it is so alien to the child's intuitive understanding about what love should look like. Finally, all of these approaches miss the best opportunities for learning because they sidetrack the child into fantasies of revenge, and he becomes too distracted to focus on the issue at hand. Real alternatives to punishment are those that help the child to learn and to grow in a healthy way.

Here are ten alternatives that give the child positive, loving messages.

1. **Prevent unwanted behavior from occurring by meeting your child's needs when they are first expressed.** This is perhaps the best approach. It not only prevents misbehavior, but it also tells the child that you truly love and care for her. With her current needs met, she is free to move on to the next stage of learning.

2. **Provide a safe, child-friendly environment.** Why have precious items within the reach of a toddler, when they can be put away until the child is old enough to handle them carefully? For older children, provide opportunities for active play.

3. **Apply the Golden Rule.** Think about how you would like to be treated if you were to find yourself in the same circumstances as your child, then treat your child that way. Human nature is human nature, regardless of age.

4. **Show empathy for your child's feelings.** Even if the child's behavior seems illogical, the underlying feelings and needs are real and need to be taken seriously. Saying things like "You really look unhappy" is a good way to show a child that you care about his needs and feelings.

5. **Validate your child's feelings.** Make sure your child knows that you understand and care, that it is acceptable to have whatever feelings are present, and that he will never be rejected for having any particular kinds of

feelings. For example, "I remember how frustrated that made me feel when I was little."

6. **Meet the underlying need that led to the behavior in the first place.** If we punish the outward behavior, the still unmet need will continually resurface in other ways until it is finally met. You may need to dig to discover what that need is. For example, your child may be feeling sad because a friend moved away, and this sadness could lead to "misbehavior."

Whenever possible, find a "win-win" solution that meets everyone's needs.

7. **Stay on your child's side.** Whenever possible, find a "win-win" solution that meets everyone's needs. To learn conflict resolution skills, consider a course in Nonviolent Communication[SM].[1]

8. **Reassure your child that she is loved and appreciated.** "Bad" behavior is often the child's attempt to express her need for more love and attention in the best way she can at that moment. If she could express this need in a more mature way, she would do so. For example, you might ask, "Would you like to read a book with me so we can have some time together?"

9. **Provide positive alternative experiences and productive activities.** Offer crayons, read a story, put a young child in the tub for water play, or enjoy a walk outside together. This can shift the focus away from a situation that has become too stressful to resolve at that moment.

10. **Ask yourself "Will I look back at this later and laugh?"** If so, why not laugh now? Seize the opportunity to create the kind of memory you will want to have when you look back on this day. The most challenging situations can be defused by the timely use of good-natured

humor. For example, "Oh, no, you and your brother painted each other green? Wait, let me get the camera!"

By keeping these alternatives in mind, we can bring about the genuine cooperation that we seek. But our greatest reward will be a lifelong, mutually loving and trusting bond with our child.

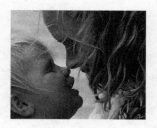

HELPING
CHILDREN LEARN

Nurturing Children's Natural Love of Learning

A s a homeschooling parent, I have often wondered who learns more in our family, the parent or the child. The topic I seem to be learning the most about is the nature of learning itself. In fact, many of the assumptions about learning found in public school teaching are reversed in homeschooling.

The main element in successful homeschooling is *trust*. We trust children to know when they are ready to learn and what they are interested in learning. We trust them to know how to go about learning. While this may seem to be an astonishing way of looking at children, parents commonly take this view of learning during the child's first two years, when he is learning to stand, walk, talk, and to perform many other important and difficult tasks with little help from anyone.

> *The main element in successful homeschooling is trust.*

No one worries that a baby will be too lazy, uncooperative, or unmotivated to learn these things; it is simply assumed that every baby is born wanting to learn what he needs to know in order to understand and to participate in

113

the world around him. These one- and two-year-old experts teach us several principles of learning:

- **Children are naturally curious and have a built-in desire to learn first-hand about the world around them.** John Holt, in his book *How Children Learn*, describes the natural learning style of young children:

    The child is curious. He wants to make sense out of things, find out how things work, gain competence and control over himself and his environment, and do what he sees other people doing. He is open, perceptive, and experimental. He does not merely observe the world around him, he does not shut himself off from the strange, complicated world around him, but tastes it, touches it, hefts it, bends it, breaks it. To find out how reality works, he works on it. He is bold. He is not afraid of making mistakes. And he is patient. He can tolerate an extraordinary amount of uncertainty, confusion, ignorance, and suspense .... School is not a place that gives much time, or opportunity, or reward, for this kind of thinking and learning.[1]

- **Children know best how to go about learning something.** If left alone, children will know instinctively what method is best for them. Caring and observant parents soon learn that it is safe and appropriate to trust this knowledge. Such parents say to their baby, "Oh, that's interesting! You're learning how to crawl downstairs by facing backwards!" They do not say, "That's the wrong way." Perceptive parents are aware that there are many different ways to learn something, and they trust their children to know which ways are best for them.

- **Children need plentiful amounts of quiet time to think.** Research shows that children who are good at fantasizing are better learners and cope better with disappointment than those who have lost this ability. But fantasy requires time, and time is the most endangered commodity in our lives. Fully scheduled school hours and extracurricular activities leave little time for children to dream, to think, to invent solutions to problems, to cope with stressful experiences, and simply to fulfill the universal need for solitude and privacy.

- **Children are not afraid to admit ignorance and to make mistakes.** When Holt invited toddlers to play his cello, they eagerly attempted to do so; school-children and adults invariably declined. Homeschooled children, free from the intimidation of public embarrassment and failing marks, retain their openness to new exploration. Children learn by asking questions, not by answering them. Toddlers ask many questions, and so do schoolchildren — until about Grade 3. By that time, many of them have learned an unfortunate fact: that in school it can be more important for self-protection to hide one's ignorance about a subject than to learn more about it, regardless of one's curiosity.

- **Children take joy in the intrinsic values of whatever they are learning.** There is no need to motivate children through the use of extrinsic rewards, such as high grades or stars. These suggest to the child that the activity must be difficult or unpleasant, otherwise why is a reward, which has nothing to do with the matter at hand, being offered? The wise parent says, "You're really enjoying that book!" not "If you read this book, you'll get a cookie."

- **Children learn best about getting along with other people through interaction with those of all ages.** No parents would tell their baby, "You may only spend time with those children whose birthdays fall within six months of your own. Here's another two-year-old to play with. You can look at each other, but no talking!" John Taylor Gatto, New York State Teacher of the Year, contends, "It is absurd, and anti-life to ... sit in confinement with people of exactly the same age and social class. That system effectively cuts you off from the immense diversity of life."[2]

- **A child learns best about the world through first-hand experience.** No parent would tell her toddler, "Let's put that caterpillar down and get back to your book about caterpillars." Homeschoolers learn directly about the world. The term "homeschooling" is misleading. Homeschooled children do not spend all of their time at home, nor is their learning approached in the same way that it would be in school. My son once described homeschooling as "learning by doing instead of being taught." Ironically, the most common objection about homeschooling is that children are "being deprived of the real world."

- **Children need and deserve ample time with their family.** Gatto warns us, "Between schooling and television, all the time children have is eaten up. That's what has destroyed the American family."[3] Many homeschoolers feel that family cohesiveness is perhaps the most meaningful benefit of the experience. Just as I saw his first step and heard his first word, I have had the honor and privilege of sharing my son's world and thoughts. Over the years I have discovered more from him about life, learning, and love than from any other source. Homeschooling is always a two-way street.

- **Stress interferes with learning**. Einstein wrote, "It is a very grave mistake to think that the enjoyment of seeing and searching can be promoted by means of coercion."[4] When a one-year-old falls down while learning to walk, we say, "Good try! You'll catch on soon!" No caring parent would say, "Every baby your age should be walking. You'd better be walking by Friday!" Most parents understand how difficult it is for their children to learn something when they are rushed, threatened, or given failing grades. John Holt warned that "we think badly, and even perceive badly, or not at all, when we are anxious or afraid ... when we make children afraid, we stop learning dead in its tracks." [4]

While infants and toddlers teach us many principles of learning, schools have adopted quite different principles due to the difficulties inherent in teaching a large number of same-age children in a compulsory setting. The structure of school (required attendance, school-selected topics and books, and constant checking of the child's progress) assumes that children are not natural learners, but must be compelled to learn through the efforts of others.

Natural learners do not need such a structure. The success of self-directed learning (homeschoolers regularly outperform their schooled peers on measures of academic achievement, socialization, confidence, and self-esteem) strongly suggests that structured approaches inhibit both learning and personal development.

Homeschooling is one attempt to follow the principles of natural learning and to help children retain the curiosity, enthusiasm, and love of learning that every child has at birth. Holt writes that homeschooling is a matter of faith:

> *This faith is that by nature people are learning animals. Birds fly; fish swim; humans think and learn. Therefore, we do not need to motivate children into learning by wheedling, bribing, or bullying. We do not need to keep picking away at their minds to make sure they are learning. What we need to do — and all we need to do — is to give children as much help and guidance as they need and ask for, listen respectfully when they feel like talking, and then get out of the way. We can trust them to do the rest.[5]*

When does Guidance become Manipulation?

M ANY HOMESCHOOLING PARENTS have puzzled over the distinction between "guidance" and "manipulation." As a parent strongly committed to "unschooling" (learner-directed homeschooling) with my son Jason, I sometimes wondered if I should encourage certain activities in spite of his lack of interest, or at least remind him of areas he had ignored for a while. This would often happen after I had heard or read of an unusually dedicated child who had excelled in a particular field of activity, such as music. It was at those times that John Holt, through his inspiring books, reminded me that trust is the most essential ingredient of a homeschooling program.

Children are surrounded by information of all kinds, through conversations, books, television, films, the Internet, stores, and nature. One day when Jason was five, he asked me about opera. This surprised me, as we had never discussed this topic. I asked what had led to his question, and he told me it had been a Bugs Bunny cartoon. He asked me several questions about types of operas, and we had a brief discussion. In spite of my own lack of interest in this subject, I trusted him to know if and when he would want more information. He knew that our encyclopedia had articles on opera and that he could find additional information at the library or from knowledgeable people. (These days, of course, virtually every topic is also covered on the Internet.)

While modeling by the parent can be helpful, if the interest the parent shows is not sincere, it will have little value. I would never feign an interest in opera or anything else. Over the years I have often seen Jason study subjects at great depth despite my own lack of interest, and I trust him to set his own "curriculum" in this way.

A subject either "clicks" with Jason, or it does not — who knows why? Initially, art, astronomy, math, and physics "clicked" strongly; over the years he has studied other areas as well. What would we have gained if I required him to study those other areas sooner? Most likely he would have felt resentment, frustration, and even less interest in those areas. If I can trust him to know what he needs to learn, and when he needs to learn it, he may some day become interested in the areas he has "missed," and with that inner motivation he can learn them quickly. Even if he "misses" a subject all his life, there should be little reason for concern. After all, no one is interested in everything, nor is every field of study essential to living a good life.

In some circumstances, we should direct and model important concepts that children may not be ready to learn all by themselves – for example, danger avoidance, constructive handling of anger, peaceful conflict resolution, compassion for others, and so on. But does Shakespeare really fit into this category? I think not, and besides, what is the rush? There seems to be an unspoken assumption in our society that if a child has not mastered each and every subject by the age of ten, we have failed in our homeschooling. But a child has a lifetime to learn whatever interests him as an adult; homeschooling advocate John Holt demonstrated this beautifully when he learned to play the cello in his 50s.

Children are adept at hearing our hidden messages. Regardless of how carefully we phrase it, when we tell a child that a certain activity is required, we imply that it must be so unpleasant or difficult that he would never want to do it on his own.

When we require a child to do something, it also implies potential punishment. If we require a certain activity, and the child is unable or unwilling to comply, then what happens? We are forced into the position of either rescinding the requirement or punishing the child. If we do nothing, we weren't really requiring the activity after all. Punishment, as discussed earlier, gives many harmful messages to the child. As Susannah Sheffer, editor of the homeschooling newsletter *Growing Without Schooling* once suggested, using force to further learning is a mistake because "it is discourteous and probably won't work anyway, and the risks of doing it are so great."[1] Perhaps one answer to the question "When does guidance become manipulation?" is "When it becomes threatening."

The goal of homeschooling is to help a child learn how to learn. At the same time, we should not dictate what that learning must be or when it must take place. As John Holt so often reminded us, the simple truth is that we can and should trust children.

School Grades: Helpful or Harmful?

The secret of education lies in respecting the pupil.
It is not for you to choose what he shall know, what
he shall do. It is foreordained, and he only holds
the key to his own secret.

— Ralph Waldo Emerson

A SCHOOL IN MY TOWN HAS offered families the option of having their children's grades given only to the parents, or to no one, on request. The children in these families would not see any grades. I believe this is a step in the right direction. However, an editorial in our local newspaper accused the parents who accepted this option of "overprotecting" their children, and preventing them from facing important consequences.

While it may be "overprotection" to hide truths from children, low grades are not "truths." Poor grades can be due to many factors beyond the child's control, such as a teacher's negative subjective impressions, the school's failure to account for individual differences, distracting family situations, misleading test questions, and false assumptions about what constitutes meaningful subject matter. Besides, if, as the editor himself suggested, children "know when they are doing well and when they are struggling," there is no need for grades. The only function a grade should have is to inform: the most useful information is whether the educational approach being used by the teacher is the appropriate one for that particular child's current interests and learning style.

A child's self-esteem is a precious commodity. Parents who attempt to maintain their child's self-esteem by avoiding the potential hazards of an imperfect, misleading, and harmful grading system should be commended, not criticized. Threatening a child with punishment for poor grades poses a danger, not just to a child's self-esteem and motivation, but also to the child's opportunity to learn in a climate that enhances learning. Tragically, the indignity of low grades, which are notoriously subjective, can effectively stop a child's learning by destroying his motivation and his belief in his own worth and abilities. School vandalism is often related to the anger and humiliation a child feels after receiving low grades. Even high grades give children the false message that extrinsic rewards are more important than the intrinsic value of learning itself. As Albert Einstein once observed, "The value of achievement lies in the achieving."

Every teaching situation involves the school, the teacher, the student, the student's parents, and the student's personal situation, among many other factors; it seems unfair and unrealistic to present low grades as a measure of the child's actions alone. Schools try to have it both ways, by taking credit when things are going well, and blaming the child, or the child's parents, when they are not.

It is ultimately the parents' right to decide whether grades are helpful or harmful for their child; after all, it is a legal option in all states and provinces in North America, and in many other countries, for children to learn at home and avoid grades entirely. For those parents considering this alternative, and for all those interested in the nature of learning, I highly recommend John Holt's fascinating book *How Children Learn*.

According to historians, Einstein kept a sign on the wall of his office: "Not everything that counts can be counted, and not everything that can be counted counts." Consider each of these phrases:

- **"Not everything that counts can be counted."** I have a friend who has more wisdom, compassion, understanding, and creativity than anyone else I know. She can see solutions to problems when no one else can and presents them with warmth and tact. She inspires many with her example of joyous living. Although she is by far the best advisor I know, she has no letters after her name. If she wanted to work as a psychologist, she would need to embark on a lengthy university course.

- **"Not everything that can be counted counts."** I have also known incompetent and uncaring health professionals who can't hold a candle to my friend, but whose professional degrees instill false confidence in their clients. They can tack a diploma to the wall, but they cannot respond from the heart. True wisdom does not come from books, nor can it be measured by tests, grades, and degrees. It comes, always, from the love one receives as a child, and from openness to the lessons life brings.

Nothing interferes with learning as much as fear — fear of poor grades, fear of parental disappointment or anger, and fear of failure. Nothing encourages learning more than the freedom to follow one's interests. Yet how can we give children this freedom while threatening them with tests and grades, ignoring their current interests, disregarding their individual approaches to learning, and ignoring their unique developmental rates? We continue to label them as "successful" or "unsuccessful" on the basis of tests that do little more than measure short-term memory, while ignoring what is truly valuable and precious within each child. This unfortunate situation, which has lasted for too many years already, needs to be addressed by school administrators, teachers, and everyone else who is concerned about the welfare of children in our world.

Nothing encourages learning more than the freedom to follow one's interests.

If the harmful nature of the competitive school grading system is recognized, and real changes are made within our schools, every child could be appreciated and valued on his or her own merits. Let's start to count what really matters.

Should Homeschoolers be Tested?

THE ASSUMPTION THAT HOMESCHOOLING parents somehow lack awareness of their children's progress, and
therefore require formal evaluation of that progress, is related to the fact that homeschoolers function beyond the arena
of the schools, and our philosophies and methods are not
always well understood. Implicit in legislators' concerns
about homeschooling students are two questions.

1. How do homeschooling parents know their children are learning?

The answer to this question is, to put it most simply, direct
observation. I have only one child. If a teacher had only one
child in her classroom and was unable to describe the reading skills of that child, everyone would be dismayed — how
could a teacher have such close daily contact with one child
and miss something so obvious? Yet many people unfamiliar
with homeschooling imagine that parents who have close
daily contact with their child require outside evaluation to
determine that child's progress. This puzzles homeschooling parents, who cannot imagine missing anything so
interesting as the nature of their child's learning.

No homeschooling parents have 25 children, so we are free to focus on the enhancement of learning without being continually distracted by the many time-consuming tasks unrelated to learning that are necessary in a classroom situation. This freedom from distraction is a major factor in the establishment of a lively, creative, and joyful learning environment.

Any parent of a preschool child could almost certainly tell us how many numbers her child can count to, and how many colors he knows — not by testing, but through many hours of listening to his questions and statements and observing his behavior. In homeschooling, this type of observation simply continues on into higher ages and more complex learning.

There are many times in the course of a day when a reasonably curious child will want to know the meaning of certain printed words — in books and newspapers, on the computer or television, on board game instruction cards, on package labels, on mail that has just arrived, and so on. If this child's self-esteem is intact, he will not hesitate to ask his parents the meanings of these words. As questions of this type decrease, and as the child begins reading aloud certain words ("Look, Daddy, this package is for you!"), it seems safe to assume that reading is progressing in the direction of literacy. Outsiders may view this as somewhat imprecise, but homeschooling parents learn through experience that more specific evaluation is intrusive, unnecessary, and self-defeating.

If the government were to establish compulsory evaluation of babies to determine whether they were walking on schedule, everyone would think it absurd. We all know that healthy babies walk eventually and that it would be futile and frustrating to attempt to speed up that process; it would be as foolish as trying to speed up the blooming of a rose. All healthy rose bushes bloom when ready, all healthy babies walk when ready, and all healthy children in a family of readers read when ready — though this may be as late as 10 or 12. There is no need to speed up or measure this process.

The child's progress is not always smooth; there may be sudden shifts from one stage to the next. A formal evaluation given just prior to such a shift may therefore give unfair and misleading information. At a time when I knew (through a reduction in the number of requests for me to read certain signs, labels, etc.) that my son Jason's reading was improving, but not yet fluent, I told him one evening that I was unable to read to him because I wasn't feeling well. He said, "Well, you can rest and I'll read a book to you." He proceeded to read an entire book flawlessly, at a level of difficulty higher than I would have guessed.

Sometimes, as in this example, in the natural course of living with a child we receive direct and specific information about his progress. But this is part of the natural process of "aiding and abetting" a child's learning, and it is almost always self-defeating to require such direct proof. Had I asked Jason to read the book, he might well have refused because he would have felt the anxiety that anyone feels when being evaluated. But because he chose to read voluntarily and his accuracy was not being examined, anxiety was not a factor.

Homeschooling parents, then, cannot help but have a good general idea of a child's progress in reading or any other area. Without testing for specific learning we may underestimate a child's abilities to some extent, but all that means is that we make delightful discoveries along the way.

2. If homeschooling parents do not measure, evaluate and control learning, how can the child himself know when to move on to the next level?

If we were to ask a horticulturist how a rose knows when to bloom, he or she could not answer that question; it is taken on faith that such knowledge is built into the miraculous design of the seed. A child's schedule of intellectual growth, like the rose's blooming, may indeed be a mysterious process, but it nonetheless exists, built into each child at conception. There is no need to impose such a process from the outside, and no one but the child has direct access to this process. Any imposition of an artificial structure will be less successful than simply leaving these determinations to the child. Any attempt to make these determinations from the outside represents guesswork that is unlikely to match the actual unfolding of interests and abilities within the child.

many homeschooling parents have reported just this sort of creativity and joyful learning in their children.

Jason, though somewhat "late" in walking (17 months) and fluent reading (7 years), one day at age three taught himself squares and square roots. How could I have guessed that he was ready for that level of mathematics on that particular day? Had I been imposing a standard curriculum, I might have discouraged early mathematics and emphasized reading, and to what end? He is now proficient in, and greatly enjoys, both areas. Ultimately, it made no difference that he achieved this mastery along unevenly timed routes. As John Holt observed, children are not trains. If a train does not reach every station on time, it will be late reaching its ultimate destination. But a child can be late at every "station" and can even change the entire route of the learning process and still reach mastery of all areas of learning in good time.

The homeschooling child knows not only what he needs to learn, but also how best to go about learning it. Jason has always devised ingenious ways for learning what is currently in the foreground of his interest. His method for learning squares and square roots — rows and columns of dots on paper — would never have occurred to me, even if I had guessed that he was ready for this subject at that early age. At about age six he was looking over a new globe and made a game pairing countries and guessing which was larger in area, then larger in population, and so on. These sorts of games went on constantly; his creativity in designing interesting learning methods far surpassed my own, and I never had to give a single thought to motivation. My child is not unique; many homeschooling parents have reported just this sort of creativity and joyful learning in their children.

Jason has had no lessons in the conventional sense. He has taught himself reading, writing, math, and science with help as needed and requested by him. However, these subjects are not treated as separate categories, but as parts of the topic of current interest. My role has been of facilitator rather than teacher, but I am not merely a passive observer. When he asked questions — which he did many times each day — I answered them as well as I could. If I didn't know the answers, I became a researcher: I made phone calls, helped him use the encyclopedia, accompanied him to the library, or found someone with relevant experience who could help him find the answer or learn about the topic. This not only answered his specific questions, but also modeled the many ways in which he could obtain information.

Regardless of which specific topics were covered, our larger curriculum has always been "how to learn" and "how to obtain information."

In the Information Age, it is no longer meaningful or realistic to require rote memorization of specific facts. These facts are not only meaningless to the child unless they happen to coincide with his own current and unique interests, but they are also simply too numerous, and many will be outdated by the time he is an adult. If a child learns how to obtain information, however, he can apply that skill throughout his life.

While we are not homeschooling for religious reasons, we have always welcomed the opportunity to explore questions of personal ethics, and to encourage such qualities as kindness, honesty, trust, cooperation, creativity (especially when it comes to solving problems), and compassion for others. This is a significant part of our "curriculum." We have also appreciated having time in the morning to discuss dreams from the previous night and to make plans for the day ahead, when I would otherwise have been preoccupied with helping Jason get ready for school. Believing that modern life is already overly hectic, we try as far as possible to make room for unhurried time in our family.

What I have described above is sometimes called "unschooling," which means the child's current interests determine the curriculum, and the parents act not as teachers but as tutors and resource assistants. This method, one of several homeschooling approaches, is often misunderstood because it is based on assumptions that are quite different from those implicit in conventional schooling. Unschoolers are more often described by what we do not do:

- We do not "teach"
- We do not impose an arbitrary, artificial curriculum
- We do not structure the hours of our "school day."

What do we do?

- We answer questions. Many of us believe that this is the most essential and critical aspect of a successful homeschooling program.
- We encourage creative and cooperative solutions to problems as they arise.
- We seek out resources and information to support whatever current interests our child is exploring.
- We attempt to illustrate, through the daily decisions we make, the benefits of such personal moral qualities as friendship, honesty, and responsibility.
- We model the joys of learning through our own discussions, reading, and research.

While it is not impossible for a family whose children go to public school to pursue the kinds of activities I have described, it is more difficult to do so when parents and children have less time together, and when after-school hours are taken up with projects, homework, and other school-related demands. In addition, schoolchildren become used to seeking emotional support from peers, and this pattern is difficult to interrupt even when school is not in session.

Rather than feeling threatened by homeschoolers and unschoolers, educators would do well to see us as colleagues and sources of information on the nature of learning and motivation. After all, we spend nearly all of our waking hours observing, studying, and participating in this fascinating endeavor. Unlike schoolteachers, we also have the luxury of continuity: we observe the same child as his or her learning unfolds over many years. This helps us understand the nature of individual intellectual development over the long term.

Homeschoolers, unschoolers, and public school educators share the same goals. That we take divergent paths to these goals should be seen not as an obstacle, but as an opportunity to explore — in a cooperative spirit — the unique discoveries each path offers.

"Learning Disability:" A Rose by Another Name

IMAGINE FOR A MOMENT THAT you are visiting a plant nursery. You hear a commotion outside, so you investigate. You find a young assistant struggling with a rose bush. He is trying to force open the petals of a rose and muttering in frustration. You ask him what he is doing, and he explains, "My boss wants all these roses to bloom this week, so last week I taped all the early ones, and now I'm opening the late ones." You protest that every rose has its own schedule of blooming; it is absurd to try to slow down or speed this up. A rose will always bloom at its own best time.

Like roses, children will all bloom at their own best time if we can meet their needs

You look at the rose again and see that it is wilting. But when you point this out, he replies, "Oh, too bad, it has genetic dysbloomia. I'll have to call an expert."

"No, no!" you say. "You caused the wilting! All you needed to do was meet the flower's needs for water and sunshine and leave the rest to nature!" You can't believe this is happening. Why is his boss so unrealistic and uninformed about roses?

Such a scene would never take place in a nursery, of course, but it happens daily in our schools. Teachers, pressured by their bosses, follow official timetables, which demand that all children learn at the same rate and in the same way. Yet children are no different than roses in their development: they are born with the capacity and desire to learn, they learn at different rates, and they learn in different ways. Like roses, children will all bloom at their own best time if we can meet their needs, provide a safe, nurturing environment, and avoid imposing our doubts, anxieties, and arbitrary timetables.

My heart goes out to those children who have been "diagnosed" with ADHD (attention-deficit and hyperactivity disorder), the latest "learning disability" label. Many educators and researchers believe that these children and their families have been cruelly deceived by the use of these labels. Dr. Thomas Armstrong, a former learning disabilities specialist, changed professions when he "began to see how this notion of learning disabilities was handicapping all of our children by placing the blame for a child's learning failure on mysterious neurological deficiencies in the brain instead of on much needed reforms in our system of education."[1]

Dr. Armstrong turned instead to the concept of learning differences. He wrote *In Their Own Way*, a fascinating and practical guide to seven personal learning styles first proposed by Harvard psychologist Howard Gardner. Dr.

Armstrong urges us to abandon convenient but harmful labels such as "dyslexia" and focus on the real problem of "dysteachia." He warns that "our schools are selling millions of kids short by writing them off as underachievers, when in reality they are disabled only by poor teaching methods."[2] He explains:

> *Children get saddled with diagnostic terms such as dyslexia, dysgraphia, dyscalculia, and the like, making it sound as if they suffer from very rare and exotic diseases. Yet the word dyslexia is just Latin bafflegab for "trouble with words" .... Hundreds of tests and programs purport to identify and remediate these "neurological dysfunctions." Yet medical doctors have yet to clearly establish any measurable brain damage in the vast majority of children with these so-called symptoms. It seems clear to me after fifteen years of research and practice in the field of education that our schools are largely to blame for the failure and boredom which millions of children face ...* [3]

Are learning disorder labels the "emperor's new clothes" of the schools? Philosophers have an interesting tool called Occam's Razor, a handy device for cutting through preposterous theories. It says that the simplest theory that fits the facts of a problem is the one that should be selected.

So what are the facts? It is a fact that many school-children, mostly males, have learning difficulties. But it is also a fact that there is a group of hundreds of thousands of children in the world, both male and female, among whom this so-called genetic defect is absent: homeschoolers. In this group, learning difficulties are rare, except for those children recently in school.

If "learning disorders" are present primarily among children in school settings, the problem must lie in the learning environment of the schools, not in some mysterious, non-quantifiable "neurological disorder" within the children, or the disorders would be equally present in home-schooling children.

Are the labels "hyperactive," "school phobic," and "learning disabled" smokescreens to hide the school's failure to understand and conform to the actual process of learning? After all, it is no secret that the schools are failing to do their job: in many areas literacy rates have actually declined and *have never reached the level they were before the existence of public schools.* When John Gatto, a New York State Teacher of the Year, calls compulsory schooling a "twelve-year jail sentence,"[4] we know that something is terribly wrong, and that the fault is not with the children.

Educator John Holt reported in *Teach Your Own* that the president of a leading learning-disability association admitted there was "little evidence to support the disability labels." Holt warns parents of schoolchildren to "be extremely skeptical of anything the schools and their specialists may say about their children and their conditions and needs. Above all, they should understand that it is almost certainly the school itself and all its tensions and anxieties that are causing these difficulties and that the best treatment for them will probably be to take the child out of school altogether."[5]

Families who have done just that are relieved to find that their children regain the love of learning they had in their early years. Unlike schoolteachers, who see a cross section of different children each year, homeschooling parents watch learning take place within the same child over many years and learn to respect each child's unique learning style, to trust the child's personal timetable, and to recognize that mistakes are a normal and temporary part of the learning process for everyone. There is no rush, after all; many homeschoolers who did not read until age 10 or 12 nonetheless have done well in college.

This relaxed attitude on the part of homeschooling parents keeps the child's self-worth intact, makes labels irrelevant, and allows learning to take place as readily as in toddlerhood: homeschoolers regularly outperform their schooled peers on measures of academic achievement, socialization, confidence, and self-esteem. In fact, Gatto reports that "children schooled at home seem to be five or even ten years ahead of their formally trained peers in their ability to think."[6]

For many years Holt challenged schools to explain the difference between a learning difficulty (which we all experience at times) and a learning disability. He asked teachers how they distinguish between causes that lie within the learner's nervous system and those factors outside the learner — the learning environment, the teacher's explanations, the teacher, or the material. Not surprisingly, he reported that he "never received any coherent answers to these questions ... [yet] this distinction is so crucial that I don't see how we can talk usefully about the learning problems of children unless we make it."

Why are teachers so sure of the existence of widespread neurological disabilities? Perhaps they confuse cause and

effect. As Holt observes, "Teachers say 'reading must be difficult, or so many children wouldn't have trouble with it.'"
Holt argues that "it is because we assume that it is so difficult that so many children have trouble with it ... all we
accomplish by our worrying, 'simplifying', and teaching, is
to make reading a hundred times harder for children than it
need be .... We think badly, or even perceive badly, or not at
all, when we are anxious and afraid."[7]

Indeed, many researchers have found that the expectations teachers have about a child's learning abilities strongly
influence the child's academic performance. Research has
also shown a high correlation between children's anxieties
and perceptual handicaps — and shows that lowering those
anxieties (and treating food allergies, if present) greatly low-
ers the incidence of such difficulties. But we don't need
researchers and experts to tell us what is wrong. We need
only listen to the children themselves, who have tried for
years to communicate their pain, frustration, confusion, and
anger. When children are driven to addictive drugs, self-
mutilation, and suicide, they are obviously trying to
communicate something of critical importance.

Are learning difficulties, in reality, the understandable
response of normal children forced to conform to the
abnormal conditions of conventional classrooms? Have the
schools failed to see the crucial difference between actual
physical or neurological problems and common, temporary
learning errors worsened by stress? While the supposed neurological anomalies have never been identified, it isn't
difficult to locate numerous abnormal conditions in the
learning environment of the schools: fierce competition;
physical inactivity (especially difficult for boys); fragmented

topics that bear little relationship to the child's own interests and experiences; constant checking and doubting of progress; insufficient family time; few opportunities to meet people of other ages; lack of quiet time for privacy and contemplation; constant and abrupt changes of topics (preventing in-depth learning); few opportunities for a teacher's undivided attention; few opportunities to share work and ideas with classmates (a golden opportunity missed); teasing by other frustrated children; discouragement caused by self-fulfilling labels; and, above all, the indignity of being a powerless "non-person" whose legitimate needs and attempts to communicate those needs are smothered by institutional defensiveness. All of these difficulties can be avoided in homeschooling — assuming that homeschooling laws allow sufficient autonomy.

"Labeling is disabling" because children believe what we tell them. If we must label something, let it be the learning environment, not the learner. Instead of "hyperactive child," we should concern ourselves with "activity-restrictive" schools; instead of an "attention-deficient student," we ought to worry about "inspiration-deficient" classrooms or "depth-deficient" curriculum; instead of "school-phobic child," we should use honest words such as "anxious" and "frightened" (and be very careful when we look for the source of that anxiety). Using Occam's Razor, let's look for the simplest theory that fits the facts, not the most obscure and complicated one! A stressful, punitive, and threatening environment is a more than sufficient explanation for learning problems. There is no need to confuse ourselves with school 'techspeak', unproven theories, and scapegoating that serve to protect a social institution that has failed our children.

What could be done instead? McGill University professor Norman Henchey recommends that we "rethink the whole notion of compulsory schooling."[8] Henchey advocates the return to homeschooling and "other routes to adulthood ... [like] apprenticeship programs, formal and informal learning services, public service. A whole variety of things might be presented to young people."

Perhaps then we can honor each child's personal learning style and, as Armstrong urges, give children the encouragement they need in order to feel like competent, successful human beings. Children are born to learn. They deserve a safe, nurturing learning environment where they can do so in an atmosphere of patience, respect, gentleness, and trust — not threats, force, and cynicism. As Einstein reminded us years ago, "It is a very grave mistake to think that the enjoyment of seeing and searching can be promoted by means of coercion."

Children are born to learn

Is *I Love Lucy* Educational?

DURING A 1997 DEBATE IN the United States Congress about an extension of the Children's Television Act that would require licensed broadcasters to air at least three hours of "educational and informative" television per day, a *USA Today* article quoted readers' viewpoints on the definition of "educational and informative."[1] One show that caused debate among readers was *I Love Lucy*, a favorite of mine.

A Detroit reader expressed the view of many adult correspondents: "While some of life's valuable lessons may be included in shows designed primarily for entertainment, that does not qualify them as educational. Education can be fun, but it is a disciplined activity. 'I Love Lucy' just doesn't fit the bill."

The children who wrote to *USA Today* took a different stand, pointing out that *I Love Lucy* teaches valuable lessons about the consequences of one's actions. They saw Lucy Ricardo, whose escapades often backfire, as a reverse role model, and the show as something of a morality play. This is an intriguing perspective because Shakespeare's plays often included comic characters from early morality plays, and his theatrical productions, written for audiences of a broad social background, were the "popular entertainment" of the day. As author-historian Frank Wadsworth noted in his *World Book* entry on Shakespeare, "Most of the Globe Theatre's audience consisted of middle-class citizens, such as merchants and craftsmen and their wives. They went to the theater for the same reasons most people today go to the movies — to relax and to escape for a while from their cares."

Shakespeare's plays were written to entertain a mass audience, the same reason many TV sitcoms and dramas are written now. At the time they were written, his plays were definitely not considered "educational and informative," nor would they have been seen as a "disciplined activity." In his day there was even some criticism of Shakespeare as an actor-turned-writer, uneducated in traditional theatrical production. Had television been invented in Elizabethan times, it is not too far-fetched to imagine *Hamlet* as one of the first TV dramas, criticized for its violence and passion.

Today, of course, Shakespeare's plays are considered a required part of a "disciplined education," with the unfortunate result of dissuading many students from enjoying the pleasures of his works.

Clearly the determination of whether a production is "educational" can change over time. Ultimately, any show can provide "educational and informative" material and food for thought on the thinking, fashions, roles, and lifestyles of its time. In fact, early shows like *I Love Lucy* are currently studied in university courses on American cultural history.

But is *I Love Lucy* educational in the ways that most people define that term? I have been impressed with the way parenting is presented on this show. Little Ricky is consistently treated with more love, kindness, and patience than is depicted in most current television families. From my perspective, nothing is more educational than that which promotes and models empathic parenting skills, especially as this essential topic is not included in most school curricula.

My son believes he has learned a great deal from *I Love Lucy* over the years. We have had many conversations about the show, covering some of the following topics:

- A good show requires skilled writers.
- Talented actors can improvise some of the best moments in a show.
- Most of the currently produced shows are more violent, less consistent in quality, and more poorly written than earlier shows.
- Persistence (such as Lucille Ball's insistence that Desi be her co-star) can bring about success.
- Smoking was common in the 1950s and not well understood.

- Marital roles have changed over the decades.
- An actor's personal life can be very different from the role he or she plays.
- If you look into history, you can sometimes discover where social changes may have been introduced (such as the three episodes in which Little Ricky is permitted to join his parents in bed when he needed emotional support).
- Even loving couples may not be able to sustain a marriage.

I could go on and on.

The indisputable point is that children are born with an insatiable curiosity. We do a real disservice when we teach a child that only some things are "educational." This always backfires anyway, as children receive the unintended but unavoidable message that the "educational" topic being presented must be difficult, dull, and something they would never want to investigate on their own, otherwise why is it being forced on them? Perhaps the most non-educational thing we can do is to convince children that "education" equals "dreariness." Children know intuitively that learning should be fun. As long as we trust this process and avoid destroying their curiosity with doubts and threats and stuffy definitions of what is "educational" and what is not, children will continue to learn from every experience they have. Any arbitrary division of the child's experiences into "entertainment" and "education" is inaccurate, misleading, self-defeating, and ultimately harmful.

> *children are born with an insatiable curiosity*

It may be that more people enjoyed Shakespeare when they were told his plays were "entertainment" than do now that the plays are held up as "educational." Let us hope the same thing never happens to Lucy.

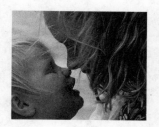

ADVOCATING FOR CHILDREN

Is There Room for Children in our Society?

MOST OF OUR CULTURE IS structured for adults, and children are often unwelcome or even excluded. Children spend most of their time in school and school-related activities, where parents are not welcome. Years ago, when my young son and I looked for activities to do together, he was told that he didn't need me, and I was told to be glad for some time alone. That we were good friends who simply wanted to enjoy an activity together was never considered.

This harsh attitude toward children is most evident when shopping. Many store personnel seem to view every child as a potential source of trouble. Children are tolerated — as long as they are perfectly quiet, don't touch anything, and don't look as though they'll hurt themselves. I suspect that it isn't so much the child's potential suffering that storekeepers are concerned about, but rather their own: they are afraid of being sued. This fear can be unreasonable to the point of lunacy. My son, at age seven, was loudly warned in a bookstore, "Get down from that ledge! You'll hurt yourself!" This dangerous ledge was a mere five inches from the floor.

When we look closely at children playing, we can see that they have the same instinct for self-preservation that adults have and a good sense of what they can handle. Why, then, are children so mistrusted?

At those times when something does need to be said about a child's behavior in public, it is likely to be done in a harsh, impatient, and disapproving tone. Yet adults too sometimes behave inappropriately in public — smoking in a non-smoking area, for example. If an adult is corrected at all, such a request is usually made with the utmost cordiality. Do adults deserve more consideration than children do?

When children venture out in public, they are rarely spoken to unless, like soldiers, they are asked their name and grade.

If children appear in public during school hours, they are asked, almost crossly, "Why aren't you in school?" How would an adult respond if asked, "Why aren't you at work?"

Children are expected to be infinitely patient during boring errands and conversations. They must never interrupt adults — no matter that children's conversations can be far and away more fascinating. What could be more interesting than hearing a detailed description of "Planet Wonderful" or learning that one is loved "Infinity squared," as my son told me when he was three?

Despite their delightful ways, children in public places are treated as though they are invisible, and their needs are often considered irrelevant. They are at a particular disadvantage when they must make their needs known to others. Who has not seen a distraught infant or child whose tears are ignored by angry parents and indifferent strangers? If an adult were crying in public, wouldn't everyone be concerned? If an animal were obviously suffering, would everyone walk past?

Churches, while teaching of love within families, segregate children from the most meaningful activities. Housing discrimination against families is still a problem in many areas, where children are placed in the same category of undesirables as pets, presumably ranking somewhere between a parakeet and a boa constrictor.

Could things be different? Things *are* different, in other cultures. When my son (age five) and I visited a Chinese herbalist, I was ignored, while the three shopkeepers, all Chinese, showered him with affectionate attention. (They did ask me one question: Did I have any more children?) Needless to say, my son felt fully accepted and appreciated, and his behavior in that store was impeccable.

All children behave as well as they are treated — just like adults. Why is it so difficult for adults to understand this? After all, we have all been children! How have we forgotten so soon what it is like to be a child in an adult world? As physicist and author Richard Feynman wrote, "Human beings should be treated like human beings." We are all human beings, and, in a sense, we are all children. Some of us have just been around a little longer.

> *All children behave as well as they are treated — just like adults.*

Intervening on Behalf of a Child
in a Public Place

S HE IS ADORABLE, ABOUT THREE, with a mass of brown curls and large blue eyes. She has just learned about pockets. She reaches out to take a small item from a shelf and holds it over her pocket. She studies the item for a moment and then lets it fall into her pocket. Plop! She gives a satisfied little laugh. She reaches into her pocket to try this again. But this is inside a store, and the item — which costs a quarter — has not been paid for.

Her father, standing nearby, has been watching this incident with growing fury. Enraged, he rushes over to the little girl, snatches the object from her hand, and shouts at her, "If you ever steal something again, I'll break your fingers!" The horror of this threat collides with her laughter, and she stands there, cowering, silent, and afraid.

This scene is, unfortunately, not fiction. It took place in a large department store in a Canadian city. It may be an extreme example, but it is not unique. We see it everywhere. A tired parent, at the end of a stressful day, loses it — and a child suffers. Many children are physically and emotionally abused every day, and we do not need to be out in public long before hearing threats, impatient commands, statements of mistrust, and angry words directed at children, and deaf ears turned to crying infants.

We'd like to help if we could, but we hesitate. Is it our business to intervene? And if we do, will we embarrass and antagonize the parent, imperiling the child even more? Will we make the mistake of harshly telling a parent to be gentle with her children? Isn't it more tactful to walk past without comment? After all, no parent is perfect.

There seems to be a common assumption in our society that intervening on behalf of a child in a public place is necessarily hurtful and critical. But there is a world of difference between officious, hurtful criticism ("How dare you treat your child like that?") and helpful, caring intervention ("It can be really hard to meet their needs when you're so busy. Is there anything I can do to help?") There is nothing inherent in intervention that requires one to be offensive. The act of offering assistance to the parent, or comfort to the child, need have no offending qualities at all.

I have successfully intervened by offering to find a mother's groceries, helping a child pick up dropped toys, and helping a mother dress a tired toddler. All of these women were genuinely grateful, thanked me for helping, and immediately began treating their children with greater compassion. I always carry colorful stickers, which I have found can distract a tired, bored, or fussy child whose parents may be too exhausted to be patient. When the child is happier from this unexpected gift (not just the sticker, but the gentle attention and eye contact as well), the parents often relax and even feel a bit energized. We can intervene in a positive way and give the message that we care about both the parent and child.

As none of us is a perfect parent, it may be most helpful to consider what type of response we ourselves would prefer if we were observed treating our children in a less than compassionate way. From this perspective, it may be helpful to follow these four steps when encountering such a situation in a public place:

1. We need to show empathy for the parent: "It can really be challenging when children are little and still learning about stores."

2. We might then share something of our own — or our child's — experience: "I remember when I was four and my parents saw me pick something up, but I didn't really understand about stealing."

3. We should then empathize with the child: "It must frighten you to see your father get so angry." We can then add: "This is a nice toy. It must be hard for you to have to leave it here."

4. Finally, we can offer a suggestion: "My child finds it helpful to keep a wish list for things we can't buy yet. You might find that helpful, too."

While it may be difficult to think of the perfect response in the heat of the moment, the sheer act of standing up for the child can have a significant impact on the child herself, even if the intervention causes the parent to become angry or defensive. Many adults in counseling sessions still recall vividly, and with gratitude, the one time that a stranger stepped in on their behalf, and how much that meant — that someone cared, and that the child's feelings of fear, confusion, and anger were understood and accepted. These adults have stated to me (and to other psychologists) that this one intervention changed their lives and gave them hope. Are we to bypass the opportunity to make such a profound difference in the life of a child?

It might help to imagine how we would act if we came upon a close friend in a similar situation. We would assume the best, that this situation was atypical and related to a stressful time in the parent's life. The first step — expressing empathy for the parent — will maximize our chances of being heard and show the parent that we believe in his good intentions. This approach offers us the best chance to avoid antagonizing the parent into further abusive behavior.

the sheer act of standing up for the child can have a significant impact on the child herself

Even in the unfortunate — and hopefully rare — case where parents are offended, the intervention may still act as a reminder that they should be more attentive to the nature of their interactions with their child. In a quieter moment, they may remember and reconsider what they were unable to accept at the time.

Intervention can be difficult, especially in a society where there are taboos against commenting on a stranger's parenting skills. For this reason, even those adults who recognize abusive treatment and empathize with the child may choose to pass by in silence. Unfortunately, walking past a distraught child also gives a message. It tells the child that no one cares about her suffering, and it implies to the parents that we approve of their behavior.

I don't advocate intervention in every case of potential abuse — I don't intervene when a child merely looks sad, for example. Babies cry for many reasons; we should not assume that the parent is at fault when we only have circumstantial evidence. Even if a baby is crying for mysterious reasons, however, the parent might welcome an offer of assistance. A simple offer to help, spoken pleasantly, is nonjudgmental and, in my experience, always welcomed. How unfortunate that the taboo against public intervention has prevented parents from helping each other in stressful situations.

On the other hand, my friends and I have witnessed some really harmful acts: slapping, hitting, shoving, arm-yanking, pinning against a wall, severe verbal abuse, negative labeling, hurtful comparisons to siblings, and so on. The children accepted this treatment because they were too helpless and inexperienced to stand up for themselves. Should we, who are older and wiser, simply walk past an obviously abusive situation? At exactly what point should we step in? Should we wait until the child is the victim of a severe physical assault? But assault takes many forms. Emotional abuse leaves no outward scars, but it still hurts children. Those of us who can recognize damaging treatment have an obligation to step in — in a compassionate and helpful way.

Psychiatric case histories clearly show that today's psychopathic adults were yesterday's hurt children. We cannot take a time machine back to help yesterday's children, but we can help today's children to become secure and responsible adults who will treat their own children with dignity, love, and compassion. We can "bear witness" in public to the children. We can let them know we value them and that we do not believe they should be mistreated. If the community does not make it clear that child abuse is unacceptable, abusive practices will only continue from one generation to the next. If we are careful to intervene in a way that shows empathy for the parent as well, we have done the job we intended.

Although the father in our story meant to give his daughter a worthwhile moral lesson, ironically his reaction is certain to lower her self-esteem and make actual theft a real possibility. How could the little girl know that his words were only a threat no sane person would carry out? The little girl's fingers were not touched, but her vision of the world she lives in will never be the same. Perhaps one day someone will come forward and speak out on her behalf — and do it so that her father can also hear the words.

Intervention can Save Lives

STATISTICALLY, IT IS RARE — far more rare than we suppose. But it is every parent's worst nightmare: a child is abducted by a stranger and never seen again. Such an event can happen in broad daylight, in a public place — a park, a shopping mall, or a neighborhood street. What can we do to prevent such a tragedy?

1. We should never assume that the adult walking with a child is, in fact, the child's parent or caretaker. If a child were being kidnapped, what would such a situation look like? Most likely we would see a child crying and struggling to get away. Unfortunately, we have all become inured to a child's cries and struggles, because children's tears and protests are often not taken seriously in our society. Yet how else would a child in this situation respond?

2. We need to teach all children exactly what the word "stranger" means. Informal surveys show that many, if not most, children believe that strangers are people who look dangerous and wear dark clothing or masks.[1] We need to make it clear that a stranger is simply *someone they do not know*. A stranger can look normal, appear friendly, and be well-dressed.

3. We can teach children to be skeptical of typical ruses used by kidnappers, such as asking the child for help.

4. Every child should have a secret code word he can ask for if someone (even someone he knows) claims a parent has sent them to pick up the child.

5. We need to teach older children to call out "This is not my mom/dad!" If the child merely cries or screams, she is likely to be ignored.

Even if what we observe is not a kidnapping, a crying child always deserves to be heard and helped. Tears and protests are a child's attempt to communicate something important. The next time you see a child whose cries are being ignored, step in. If you can respond in a caring and peaceful way, you will help ensure that a child's important message is heard. And you may even save a life.

Age Discrimination Harms
Young and Old Alike

HERE IS A RIDDLE: "I don't have much hair, I don't have all my teeth, I have trouble walking, I need help dressing myself, I am often misunderstood, and I sometimes feel unwanted. Who am I?"

If you guessed "a toddler," you are correct. If you guessed "an elderly person," right again. These two groups have much in common, but there is one important difference. Seniors have spokespeople to help make their needs known. Toddlers have no such help. When they try in the only ways they can to let us know their human rights are being violated, they are seldom taken seriously; instead they are often ridiculed or even punished.

The young and the old cannot manage all of their own physical care, and they need and deserve respectful help. My first awareness of the similarities between the very young and the very old took place in Ohio in 1982. My son Jason, his grandmother Anabel Hunt, and I were visiting Anabel's parents, then in their 80s. When it was time to leave, I found Jason's shoes and began to help him put them on. I happened to glance around the room and smiled. There was Anabel, kneeling down, tying Grandpa's shoelaces.

But the similarities go beyond physical assistance. A few years ago in my city, an 80-year-old woman, suffering from osteoporosis and arthritis, was enjoying a rare excursion downtown. Painfully stooped over, she slowly made her way down the street. At first she was ignored by the strangers she passed, and she felt lonely among the crowds. But then someone noticed her and spoke. "Look at the hunchback!" Shocked, the woman said nothing. Later, when she arrived home, she burst into tears and told the story to her son. She then added, wistfully, "They used to say I was pretty."

At an outdoor gathering I overheard a young mother scold her one-year-old: "Put on a shirt. You look stupid!"

In a grocery store, a four-year-old boy tried, unsuccessfully, to lift a heavy item his father had just selected. Instead of helping his son, the father became angry, and swore at him.

The young and the old are often criticized for things beyond their control, and they deserve our understanding. The elderly should not be blamed for their frailty and lost youth, nor should children be blamed for things they have not yet learned to do. But the similarities in the way society treats these two groups go deeper still.

Both groups find their needs shoved aside when they interfere with the needs of others. Seniors battle age discrimination in the workplace, while families battle "no children allowed" policies in housing. When either children or the elderly voice their opinions, they often find it difficult to get our attention. It is as though children are expected to "stay in their place" — at home, at school, or in day care — while the elderly are expected to "fade away" gracefully from the rest of society. When they are not in "their place," but happen to be present in a group of mixed ages, both children and the elderly are expected to be quiet, well-behaved, and non-demanding. There is something curious going on here; this is happening even though we have all been children in the past and — if we are fortunate — will be elderly in the future.

Programs for children and for seniors naturally reflect these negative attitudes and tend to meet the needs of the institutions that isolate these groups, overlooking their personal needs. More government funds are available for institutional care for the elderly than for the type of care that could enable them to remain at home, as most would wish. Similarly, legislators promise more day-care programs, rather than offering funding or tax incentives for parents that could allow babies and toddlers to remain at home, as they would wish.

Both young and old clearly deserve more choices in where and how they spend their time, and they should not be so completely at the mercy of others' decisions. Still, the need for expanded choices for seniors is more acceptable in our society than is the concept of more freedom for children, who are seen as somehow different in nature than the rest of humanity — as property rather than as human beings deserving of human rights. Indeed, many fear the whole concept of "children's rights" as a threat to parents' authority. In response to that fear, John Holt replied:

> *If I had to make a general rule for living and work-*
> *ing with children, it might be this: be very wary of say-*
> *ing or doing anything to a child that you would not*
> *do to another adult, whose good opinion and affection*

you valued. Of course, if we saw someone walking toward an open manhole or some other grave danger, we would shout, "Look out!" In this spirit we often and rightly intervene in the lives of children.

But this has almost nothing to do with "adult authority," some kind of general right and duty to tell children what to do. It would be equally right and natural if an eight-year-old I know, already an expert skier, should tell some adult that a certain trail was probably too difficult for him, and that he should stay off it. What is speaking here is not the authority of age, but the authority of greater experience and understanding, which does not necessarily have anything to do with age.[1]

It is not just eight-year-old skiers who are expert enough about a matter to give us advice; a newborn refusing a bottle is advising us — in the only way available to her — of the superiority of breastfeeding; a baby who cries when "put down" is an authority on the critical importance of bonding through touch; a child who cries in the night is communicating the wisdom of centuries of families sleeping together.

We need to free ourselves from age stereotypes and begin to appreciate and respect others of all ages. But until we reach that point, legislation and official spokespersons will be needed for young and old alike.

Rejection and mistrust of children and seniors is especially prevalent in North America; in other cultures they are more warmly welcomed and accepted. In Scandinavia, government subsidies allow the elderly to remain at home, where they receive free meals, transportation, and care; for children there are laws prohibiting spanking and bullying, requiring the initiation of breastfeeding, and even regulating the design of new buildings from a child's point of view. Norway has a Commissioner for Children — the first in the world — an independent, public spokesperson who protects children's interests.

These successful programs give us hope and set examples for the work that lies ahead. We have begun the process of legislating the rights of senior citizens, but more needs to be done. We also need to consider the rights of children, who cannot speak for themselves and who are therefore the most vulnerable group in our society.

"A person's a person, no matter how small"

As Dr. Seuss reminds us, "A person's a person, no matter how small" — or how frail. We should treat one another with love and respect, free from biases and expectations based on age. When both young and old are valued for their ageless spirit within, we will all live more freely and joyfully.

The Kids' Project: Breaking the Cycle of Abuse

ONE SUNDAY EVENING IN AUGUST 1986, Rick Lahrson of Portland, Oregon, was seated at a restaurant. He was enjoying some coffee and looking over the menu when he overheard parents berating their children. With a heavy heart he listened to the steady stream of hurtful messages and threats, the tension mounting with every word they spoke. It was clear to Lahrson that this was not a momentary lapse of patience that all parents experience. Rather, it seemed to reflect the parents' usual way of relating to their children. The three children, aged about three to six, appeared to have already lost some of their spark.

This experience was so painful that Lahrson could not order a meal and had to leave the restaurant. As he later described it, "These kids were absolutely delightful, but the parents just couldn't see it. They were suffocating the life out of these children, and it was just so wrong. I'd witnessed the same thing so often that I just couldn't take it any longer."

As he left the restaurant, he could see that the hostess was watching the scene with a frown. "Somebody has to break that cycle," Lahrson commented to her. Within a few steps he realized what he had just said and knew that he had made a personal commitment. By the fall of that year his non-profit organization, The Kids' Project, was underway, dedicated to creating a world in which children are treated with dignity and respect. Lahrson's goal was to break the cycle of child abuse by changing adults' perceptions of children. As he explained at the time, "Human beings are not born questioning their own worth. Infants have an abundance of what we call self-esteem. They are uninhibited, avid learners with no hidden agendas and no need to compensate for lost self-esteem or to covertly manipulate others."[1]

> *Loving and respectful treatment of children is critical to their future happiness and to the welfare of society as a whole.*

Lahrson hoped to bring about a transformation in our thinking and in our interactions with children so that "every man, woman, and child will be recognized as a complete, loving human being with the ability and desire to be a contribution to others. Crime, war, poverty, and fear will be things of the past."

These may sound like lofty and unrelated goals, but many psychologists believe that drug, alcohol, and nicotine dependence and sociopathic behaviors stem from the unmet needs of our earliest years. Loving and respectful treatment of children is critical to their future happiness and to the welfare of society as a whole. Yet parents who were not given love and respect in childhood have not learned how to treat others this way. Are we then locked into inadequate or abusive parenting, generation after generation? What can we as a society do to break free from this heartbreaking pattern?

Lahrson listed the following set of beliefs as a starting point for transforming our consciousness about children:

- From before birth, children have the same ability to think and to feel that adults have, minus the experience and allowing for stages of development.
- Children have a voracious appetite for learning, and they learn best the things they learn first. Children, like adults, learn mostly by example and experience.
- Children have a drive to love other people and to give of themselves to the people around them.
- Children offer a joyful zest for life and a fresh point of view.
- Children are empirical scientists of the first order. A child's logic is flawless, based on his or her experience and stage of development.

- Children are frequently misunderstood in their early communications and are often squelched, rather than listened to fairly.
- Misbehavior in children is an attempt to communicate when all else has failed.

As John Holt wrote, "All I am saying can be summed up in two words: 'trust children'. Nothing could be more simple — or more difficult. Difficult, because to trust children we must trust ourselves — and most of us were taught as children that we could not be trusted."[2]

Our interpretation of a child's intentions will have a significant effect on our relationship with them and their own view of themselves. If we believe our child's intentions are good, it will lead to an upward spiral of good will: the more we trust the child, the more loving and cooperative he becomes, and the easier it becomes for us to trust him in the future.

Conclusion

THERE IS A FRENCH SAYING, "Tout comprendre, c'est tout pardonner, which translates "To know all is to forgive all". Clarence Darrow, the famous 19th Century lawyer, took this a step further: "To know all is to understand all, and this leaves no room for judgment or condemnation."

When we believe in our child fully, we trust that they are doing the very best they can at every moment, given their age, past experience and present circumstances. It is this kind of trust that I mean when I talk about parents being on their child's side. Having someone dependably "on their side" is absolutely critical if a child is to grow into adulthood with a generous capacity for love and trust.

If we aren't on their side, who will be?

Endnotes

"Getting It" About Children

1. Marshall Rosenberg, *Nonviolent Communication: A Language of Compassion* (Encinitas, California: PuddleDancer Press, 2000).

2. Elliott Barker, Editorial in *Empathic Parenting* 23, no. 1 (2000).

The Importance of Empathic Parenting

1. Alice Miller, *Banished Knowledge: Facing Childhood Injuries*, new edition (New York: Anchor Press, 1997).

2. Elliott Barker, Film Guide to CSPCC Videotape *When You Can't Feel No Love* (Canadian Society for the Prevention of Cruelty to Children, 1991).

3. William Sears, M.D., *Creative Parenting: How to Use the Attachment Parenting Concept to Raise Children Successfully from Birth Through Adolescence* (Montreal: Optimum Publishing International, 1987).

Nature or Nurture?

1. Sidney D. Craig, *Raising Your Child, not by Force but by Love* (Philadelphia: Westminster Press, 1973).

2. "Childhood Trauma" was presented as a lecture in New York City on October 22, 1998.

Tough Love

1. John Holt quoted in "Good Times Prepare for Bad," *Growing Without Schooling*, no. 54 (December 1986).

A Baby Cries

1. See articles on crime prevention at the *Empathic Parenting* website (Canadian Society for the Prevention of Cruelty to Children), <www.empathicparenting.org/>.

2. Jean Liedloff, *The Continuum Concept: In Search of Happiness Lost*, Classics in Human Development (Reading, Massachusetts: Addison-Wesley Publishing Company Inc., 1985).

Siblings Arrive All at Once

1. Elliott Barker, Editorial in *Empathic Parenting* 23, no. 1 (2000).

Lonely Cages

1. James J. McKenna, "The Potential Benefits of Infant-Parent Cosleeping in Relation to SIDS Prevention," in *SIDS in the '90s*, edited by Torliev O. Rognum (Vancouver: Scandinavian Press, 1995).

2. James J. McKenna, personal communication, June 2000; and "Is sleeping with my baby safe? Can it reduce the risk of SIDS?" *Horizons* 1, no. 4 (spring/summer 1995).

3. "Safety Hazards in Child Care Settings" (Washington, DC: U.S. Consumer Product Safety Commission, April 1999).

4. John Holt quoted in "Good Times Prepare for Bad," *Growing Without Schooling*, no. 54 (December 1986).

Ten Ways to Grow a Happy Child

1. Ken Magid, *High Risk: Children Without a Conscience* (Bantam Books, 1989).

2. The first three points are excerpted and adapted from Elliott Barker, Film Guide to *When You Can't Feel No Love*.

3. George Wootan, "Breastfeeding: New Discoveries" on the Natural Child Project website <http://www.naturalchild.org/guest/george_wootan.html>.

4. John Valusek, "People are Not for Hitting and Children are People Too," *Empathic Parenting* 22, no. 1 (winter 1999).

5. Barker, Film Guide.

Ten Tips for Finding a Medical Professional for Your Child

1. Dr. Priscilla Alderson, "European Charter of Children's Rights," *Bulletin of Medical Ethics* No. 92 (October 1993).

The "Magic Words" Must be Spoken from the Heart

1. John Holt, *Growing Without Schooling* no. 35, p. 21.

The Trouble With Rewards

1. Mary Van Doren, personal communication, 1997.

It Shouldn't Hurt to be a Child

1. An earlier version of this article appeared as Appendix D in Alice Miller's book *Breaking Down the Wall of Silence* New York: Plume (Plume, revised edition 1997).

2. Peter Newell, personal communication, June 1991. EPOCH Worldwide is at 77 Holloway Road, London N78JZ UK. Its goals are: To see that all children will be entitled to the same protections against assault that adults now receive; to broaden the public's awareness of the harmful, long-term repercussions of physical punishment and its potential to escalate into child abuse; to provide a widespread educational program that presents and encourages positive alternative methods of gaining cooperation from children.

3. Adah Maurer in a pamphlet by End Violence Against the Next Generation (EVAN-G), 977 Keeler Avenue, Berkeley, CA 94708, USA.

4. I Corinthians 13: iv.

5. For more on this topic, see Tom Johnson, *The Sexual Dangers of Spanking Children* (Alamo, California: Parents and Teachers Against Violence in Education, 1996).

6. Adapted from Aletha Solter, "The Disadvantages of Time-Out," *Mothering* 65 (Winter 1992).

7. Elliott Barker, Editorial in *Empathic Parenting* 23, no. 1 (2000).

The Dangers of Holding Therapy

1. Martha Welch, *Holding Time* (New York: Fireside Publishers, 1989).

2. See Marshall Rosenberg's thoughtful discussion on "The Protective Use of Force" in *Nonviolent Communication: A Language of Compassion* (Encinitas, CA: Puddledancer Press, 2000).

3. S.F. Maier and M.E.P. Seligman, "Learned Helplessness: Theory and Evidence," *Journal of Experimental Psychology General* 105 (1976).

Ten Alternatives to Punishment

1. Available from the Center for Nonviolent Communication, P.O. Box 2662, Sherman, Texas 75091-2662, Tel: 903-893-3886; Fax: 903-893-2935; email: cnvc@compuserve.com.

Nurturing Children's Natural Love of Learning

1. John Holt, *How Children Learn* (New York: Delacorte Press, 1983).

2. John Gatto, "Why Schools Don't Educate," *The Sun* (June 1990).

3. Ibid.

4. Holt, *How Children Learn.*

5. Ibid.

When does Guidance become Manipulation?

1. Susannah Sheffer, "Discussion: When does guidance become manipulation?" *Growing Without Schooling* no. 75 (1990).

"Learning Disability:" A Rose by Another Name

1. Thomas Armstrong, *In Their Own Way* (New York: Putnam Publishing Group, 2000).

2. Ibid.

3. Ibid.

4. John Gatto, "The Seven Lesson School Teacher," New York City Teacher of the Year acceptance speech, New York State Senate, 1990.

5. John Holt, *Teach Your Own* (New York: Dell Publishing Co., 1981).

6. John Gatto, *Dumbing Us Down: The Hidden Curriculum of Compulsory Schooling* (Gabriola Island, BC: New Society Publishers, 1991).

7. Holt, *Teach Your Own.*

8. Norman Henchey, "Rethinking Compulsory Schooling," *Growing Without Schooling* no. 59 (October 1987).

Is *I Love Lucy* Educational?

1. *USA Today Online*, September 24, 1996.

Intervention Can Save Lives

1. Cheralyn Maturi, "Strangers: What Do They Look Like?" on the Natural Child Project website <www.naturalchild.org /guest/cheralyn_maturi.html>.

Age Discrimination Harms Young and Old Alike

1. John Holt, *Teach Your Own* (New York: Dell Publishing Co., 1981).

The Kids' Project: Breaking the Cycle of Abuse

1. Rick's statements appeared in his Kids' Project pamphlet, published in 1987.

2. John Holt, *How Children Learn* (New York: Delacorte Press, 1983).

About the Author

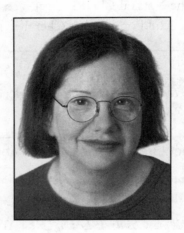

JAN HUNT, B.A. PSYCHOLOGY, M.Sc. Counseling Psychology, is the Director of the Natural Child Project and the Editorial Assistant of the quarterly journal *Empathic Parenting*, published by the Canadian Society for the Prevention of Cruelty to Children (CSPCC). She is a member of the Board of Directors for the CSPCC and The Alliance for Transforming the Lives of Children. She is also on the Advisory Board of The Child-Friendly Initiative and Attachment Parenting International and is a consultant for Northwest Attachment Parenting.

Jan's parenting column "The Natural Child" appeared in *Natural Life* from 1992 to 1999. One of her columns,

"Ten Reasons Not to Hit Your Kids" was selected as an appendix to Alice Miller's book, *Breaking Down the Wall of Silence* (New York: Penguin USA, new edition 1997). Jan is the parent of a 20-year-old son, Jason, who homeschooled from the beginning with a learner-directed approach. Jason is the webmaster for The Natural Child Project web site. Jan and her son live in Central Oregon.

See Jan's parenting advice and more articles by leading mental health professionals at The Natural Child Project at www.naturalchild.org.

The Global Children's Art Gallery displays hundreds of pictures by children age 1 to 12 from around the world at www.naturalchild.org/gallery.

If you have enjoyed *The Natural Child*, you might enjoy other

Books to Build a New Society

Our books provide positive solutions for people who want
to make a difference. We specialize in:

**Educational and Parenting Resources • Nonviolence
Sustainable Living • Ecological Design and Planning
Natural Building & Appropriate Technology • New Forestry
Environment and Justice • Conscientious Commerce
Progressive Leadership • Resistance and Community**

New Society Publishers

ENVIRONMENTAL BENEFITS STATEMENT

New Society Publishers has chosen to produce this book on New Leaf EcoBook 100,
recycled paper made with 100% post consumer waste, processed chlorine free, and
old growth free.

For every 5,000 books printed, New Society saves the following resources:[1]

18	Trees
1,587	Pounds of Solid Waste
1,746	Gallons of Water
2,278	Kilowatt Hours of Electricity
2,885	Pounds of Greenhouse Gases
12	Pounds of HAPs, VOCs, and AOX Combined
4	Cubic Yards of Landfill Space

[1]Environmental benefits are calculated based on research done by the Environmental Defense Fund and
other members of the Paper Task Force who study the environmental impacts of the paper industry.

For more information on this environmental benefits statement, or to inquire about environmentally
friendly papers, please contact New Leaf Paper – info@newleafpaper.com Tel: 888 • 989 • 5323.

For a full list of NSP's titles, please call **1-800-567-6772** *or check out our web site at:*

www.newsociety.com

New Society Publishers